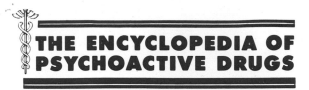
THE ENCYCLOPEDIA OF PSYCHOACTIVE DRUGS

SERIES 1

The Addictive Personality
Alcohol and Alcoholism
Alcohol Customs and Rituals
Alcohol Teenage Drinking
Amphetamines Danger in the Fast Lane
Barbiturates Sleeping Potion or Intoxicant?
Caffeine The Most Popular Stimulant
Cocaine A New Epidemic
Escape from Anxiety and Stress
Flowering Plants Magic in Bloom
Getting Help Treatments for Drug Abuse
Heroin The Street Narcotic
Inhalants The Toxic Fumes

LSD Visions or Nightmares?
Marijuana Its Effects on Mind & Body
Methadone Treatment for Addiction
Mushrooms Psychedelic Fungi
Nicotine An Old-Fashioned Addiction
Over-The-Counter Drugs Harmless or Hazardous?
PCP The Dangerous Angel
Prescription Narcotics The Addictive Painkillers
Quaaludes The Quest for Oblivion
Teenage Depression and Drugs
Treating Mental Illness
Valium and Other Tranquilizers

SERIES 2

Bad Trips
Brain Function
Case Histories
Celebrity Drug Use
Designer Drugs
The Downside of Drugs
Drinking, Driving, and Drugs
Drugs and Civilization
Drugs and Crime
Drugs and Diet
Drugs and Disease
Drugs and Emotion
Drugs and Pain
Drugs and Perception
Drugs and Pregnancy
Drugs and Sexual Behavior

Drugs and Sleep
Drugs and Sports
Drugs and the Arts
Drugs and the Brain
Drugs and the Family
Drugs and the Law
Drugs and Women
Drugs of the Future
Drugs Through the Ages
Drug Use Around the World
Legalization: A Debate
Mental Disturbances
Nutrition and the Brain
The Origins and Sources of Drugs
Substance Abuse: Prevention and Treatment
Who Uses Drugs?

DRUG USE
AROUND
THE WORLD

GENERAL EDITOR
Professor Solomon H. Snyder, M.D.

Distinguished Service Professor of
Neuroscience, Pharmacology, and Psychiatry at
The Johns Hopkins University School of Medicine

•

ASSOCIATE EDITOR
Professor Barry L. Jacobs, Ph.D.

Program in Neuroscience, Department of Psychology,
Princeton University

•

SENIOR EDITORIAL CONSULTANT
Joann Rodgers

Deputy Director, Office of Public Affairs at
The Johns Hopkins Medical Institutions

THE ENCYCLOPEDIA OF PSYCHOACTIVE DRUGS

SERIES 2

DRUG USE AROUND THE WORLD

MARC KUSINITZ

CHELSEA HOUSE PUBLISHERS
NEW YORK • NEW HAVEN • PHILADELPHIA

Chelsea House Publishers

EDITOR-IN-CHIEF: Nancy Toff
EXECUTIVE EDITOR: Remmel T. Nunn
MANAGING EDITOR: Karyn Gullen Browne
COPY CHIEF: Juliann Barbato
PICTURE EDITOR: Adrian G. Allen
ART DIRECTOR: Giannella Garrett
MANUFACTURING MANAGER: Gerald Levine

The Encyclopedia of Psychoactive Drugs

SENIOR EDITOR: Jane Larkin Crain

Staff for: DRUG USE AROUND THE WORLD

ASSOCIATE EDITOR: Paula Edelson
ASSISTANT EDITOR: Laura-Ann Dolce
COPY EDITOR: Karen Hammonds
DEPUTY COPY CHIEF: Ellen Scordato
EDITORIAL ASSISTANT: Susan DeRosa
ASSOCIATE PICTURE RESEARCHER: Juliette Dickstein
PICTURE RESEARCHER: Kim Dramer
DESIGNER: Victoria Tomaselli
ASSISTANT DESIGNER: Donna Sinisgalli
PRODUCTION COORDINATOR: Joseph Romano

First Printing

1   3   5   7   9   8   6   4   2

Library of Congress Cataloging in Publication Data

Kusinitz, Marc
  Drug Use Around the World.

  (The Encyclopedia of Psychoactive Drugs. Series 2)
  Bibliography: p.
  Includes index.
  Summary: Discusses the problems of global drug abuse, from Europe, Africa,
and the Far East to Latin America and North America.
    1. Drug abuse—Cross-cultural studies—Juvenile literature. 2. Drug abuse—
Prevention—Cross-cultural studies—Juvenile literature. [1. Drug abuse]
I. Title. II. Series.
HV5801.H63   1988   362.2'932   88-6140
ISBN 1-55546-233-2

CONTENTS

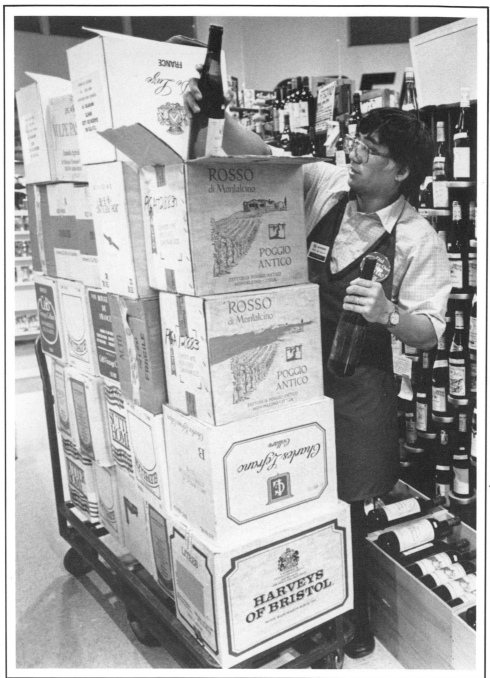

A clerk unpacks wine in a liquor store. Alcohol, which was originally used in sacred religious rituals, is now the most easily available and widely abused drug in the world.

FOREWORD

In the Mainstream
of American Life

One of the legacies of the social upheaval of the 1960s is that psychoactive drugs have become part of the mainstream of American life. Schools, homes, and communities cannot be "drug proofed." There is a demand for drugs — and the supply is plentiful. Social norms have changed and drugs are not only available—they are everywhere.

But where efforts to curtail the supply of drugs and outlaw their use have had tragically limited effects on demand, it may be that education has begun to stem the rising tide of drug abuse among young people and adults alike.

Over the past 25 years, as drugs have become an increasingly routine facet of contemporary life, a great many teenagers have adopted the notion that drug taking was somehow a right or a privilege or a necessity. They have done so, however, without understanding the consequences of drug use during the crucial years of adolescence.

The teenage years are few in the total life cycle, but critical in the maturation process. During these years adolescents face the difficult tasks of discovering their identity, clarifying their sexual roles, asserting their independence, learning to cope with authority, and searching for goals that will give their lives meaning.

Drugs rob adolescents of precious time, stamina, and health. They interrupt critical learning processes, sometimes forever. Teenagers who use drugs are likely to withdraw increasingly into themselves, to "cop out" at just the time when they most need to reach out and experience the world.

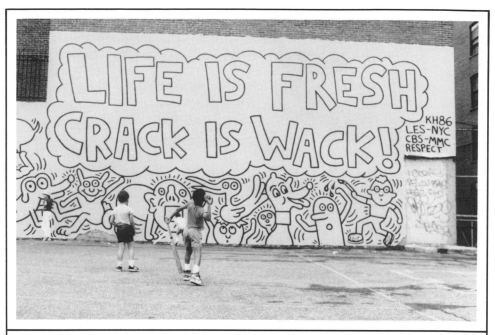

A New York City mural gives some wise advice. During the late 1980s, the sale of crack, an adulterated, deadly form of cocaine, spawned an epidemic of violence in inner cities throughout the United States.

Fortunately, as a recent Gallup poll shows, young people are beginning to realize this, too. They themselves label drugs their most important problem. In the last few years, moreover, the climate of tolerance and ignorance surrounding drugs has been changing.

Adolescents as well as adults are becoming aware of mounting evidence that every race, ethnic group, and class is vulnerable to drug dependency.

Recent publicity about the cost and failure of drug rehabilitation efforts; dangerous drug use among pilots, air traffic controllers, star athletes, and Hollywood celebrities; and drug-related accidents, suicides, and violent crime have focused the public's attention on the need to wage an all-out war on drug abuse before it seriously undermines the fabric of society itself.

The anti-drug message is getting stronger and there is evidence that the message is beginning to get through to adults and teenagers alike.

The Encyclopedia of Psychoactive Drugs hopes to play a part in the national campaign now underway to educate young people about drugs. Series 1 provides clear and comprehensive discussions of common psychoactive substances, outlines their psychological and physiological effects on the mind and body, explains how they "hook" the user, and separates fact from myth in the complex issue of drug abuse.

Whereas Series 1 focuses on specific drugs, such as nicotine or cocaine, Series 2 confronts a broad range of both social and physiological phenomena. Each volume addresses the ramifications of drug use and abuse on some aspect of human experience: social, familial, cultural, historical, and physical. Separate volumes explore questions about the effects of drugs on brain chemistry and unborn children; the use and abuse of painkillers; the relationship between drugs and sexual behavior, sports, and the arts; drugs and disease; the role of drugs in history; and the sophisticated drugs now being developed in the laboratory that will profoundly change the future.

Each book in the series is fully illustrated and is tailored to the needs and interests of young readers. The more adolescents know about drugs and their role in society, the less likely they are to misuse them.

Joann Rodgers
Senior Editorial Consultant

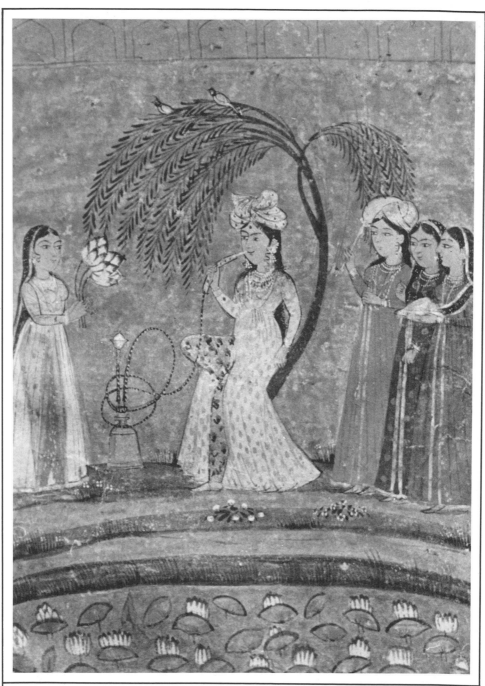

A painted miniature from a 15th-century Persian manuscript depicts a woman smoking hashish. This drug, derived from the same plant as marijuana, has been used in the Middle East for thousands of years.

INTRODUCTION

The Gift of Wizardry
Use and Abuse

JACK H. MENDELSON, M.D.
NANCY K. MELLO, Ph.D.
Alcohol and Drug Abuse Research Center
Harvard Medical School—McLean Hospital

Dorothy to the Wizard:

"I think you are a very bad man," said Dorothy.
"Oh no, my dear; I'm really a very good man; but I'm a very bad Wizard."
—from THE WIZARD OF OZ

Man is endowed with the gift of wizardry, a talent for discovery and invention. The discovery and invention of substances that change the way we feel and behave are among man's special accomplishments, and, like so many other products of our wizardry, these substances have the capacity to harm as well as to help. Psychoactive drugs can cause profound changes in the chemistry of the brain and other vital organs, and although their legitimate use can relieve pain and cure disease, their abuse leads in a tragic number of cases to destruction.

Consider alcohol — available to all and yet regarded with intense ambivalence from biblical times to the present day. The use of alcoholic beverages dates back to our earliest ancestors. Alcohol use and misuse became associated with the worship of gods and demons. One of the most powerful Greek gods was Dionysus, lord of fruitfulness and god of wine. The Romans adopted Dionysus but changed his name to Bacchus. Festivals and holidays associated with Bacchus celebrated the harvest and the origins of life. Time has blurred the images of the Bacchanalian festival, but the theme of drunkenness as a major part of celebration has survived the pagan gods and remains a familiar part of modern society. The term "Bacchanalian Festival" conveys a more appealing image than "drunken orgy" or "pot party," but whatever the label, drinking alcohol is a form of drug use that results in addiction for millions.

The fact that many millions of other people can use alcohol in moderation does not mitigate the toll this drug takes on society as a whole. According to reliable estimates, one out of every ten Americans develops a serious alcohol-related problem sometime in his or her lifetime. In addition, automobile accidents caused by drunken drivers claim the lives of tens of thousands every year. Many of the victims are gifted young people, just starting out in adult life. Hospital emergency rooms abound with patients seeking help for alcohol-related injuries.

Who is to blame? Can we blame the many manufacturers who produce such an amazing variety of alcoholic beverages? Should we blame the educators who fail to explain the perils of intoxication, or so exaggerate the dangers of drinking that no one could possibly believe them? Are friends to blame — those peers who urge others to "drink more and faster," or the macho types who stress the importance of being able to "hold your liquor"? Casting blame, however, is hardly constructive, and pointing the finger is a fruitless way to deal with the problem. Alcoholism and drug abuse have few culprits but many victims. Accountability begins with each of us, every time we choose to use or misuse an intoxicating substance.

It is ironic that some of man's earliest medicines, derived from natural plant products, are used today to poison and to intoxicate. Relief from pain and suffering is one of society's many continuing goals. Over 3,000 years ago, the Therapeutic Papyrus of Thebes, one of our earliest written records, gave instructions for the use of opium in the treatment of pain. Opium, in the form of its major derivative, morphine, and similar compounds, such as heroin, have also been used by many to induce changes in mood and feeling. Another example of man's misuse of a natural substance is the coca leaf, which for centuries was used by the Indians of Peru to reduce fatigue and hunger. Its modern derivative, cocaine, has important medical use as a local anesthetic. Unfortunately, its increasing abuse in the 1980s clearly has reached epidemic proportions.

The purpose of this series is to explore in depth the psychological and behavioral effects that psychoactive drugs have on the individual, and also, to investigate the ways in which drug use influences the legal, economic, cultural, and even moral aspects of societies. The information presented here (and in other books in this series) is based on many clinical and laboratory studies and other observations by people from diverse walks of life.

Over the centuries, novelists, poets, and dramatists have provided us with many insights into the sometimes seductive but ultimately problematic aspects of alcohol and drug use. Physicians, lawyers, biologists, psychologists, and social scientists have contributed to a better understanding of the causes and consequences of using these substances. The authors in this series have attempted to gather and condense all the latest information about drug use and abuse. They have also described the sometimes wide gaps in our knowledge and have suggested some new ways to answer many difficult questions.

One such question, for example, is how do alcohol and drug problems get started? And what is the best way to treat them when they do? Not too many years ago, alcoholics and drug abusers were regarded as evil, immoral, or both. It is now recognized that these persons suffer from very complicated diseases involving deep psychological and social problems. To understand how the disease begins and progresses, it is necessary to understand the nature of the substance, the behavior of addicts, and the characteristics of the society or culture in which they live.

Although many of the social environments we live in are very similar, some of the most subtle differences can strongly influence our thinking and behavior. Where we live, go to school and work, whom we discuss things with — all influence our opinions about drug use and misuse. Yet we also share certain commonly accepted beliefs that outweigh any differences in our attitudes. The authors in this series have tried to identify and discuss the central, most crucial issues concerning drug use and misuse.

Despite the increasing sophistication of the chemical substances we create in the laboratory, we have a long way to go in our efforts to make these powerful drugs work for us rather than against us.

The volumes in this series address a wide range of timely questions. What influence has drug use had on the arts? Why do so many of today's celebrities and star athletes use drugs, and what is being done to solve this problem? What is the relationship between drugs and crime? What is the physiological basis for the power drugs can hold over us? These are but a few of the issues explored in this far-ranging series.

Educating people about the dangers of drugs can go a long way towards minimizing the desperate consequences of substance abuse for individuals and society as a whole. Luckily, human beings have the resources to solve even the most serious problems that beset them, once they make the commitment to do so. As one keen and sensitive observer, Dr. Lewis Thomas, has said,

> There is nothing at all absurd about the human condition. We matter. It seems to me a good guess, hazarded by a good many people who have thought about it, that we may be engaged in the formation of something like a mind for the life of this planet. If this is so, we are still at the most primitive stage, still fumbling with language and thinking, but infinitely capacitated for the future. Looked at this way, it is remarkable that we've come as far as we have in so short a period, really no time at all as geologists measure time. We are the newest, youngest, and the brightest thing around.

DRUG USE AROUND THE WORLD

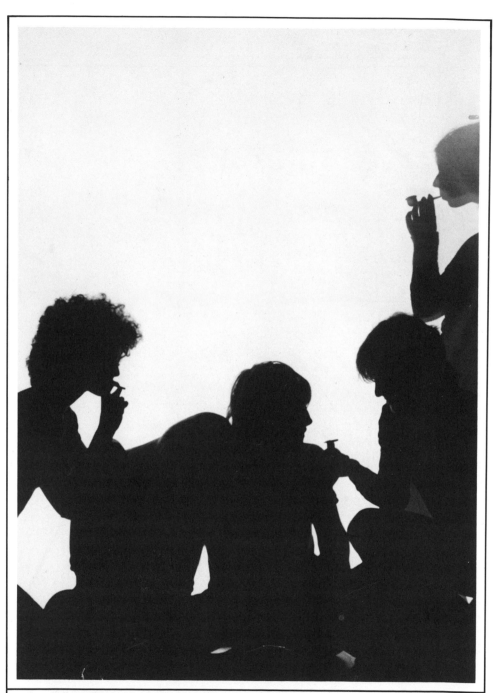

A group of boys smoking marijuana. The perception of what constitutes drug abuse varies from culture to culture and from generation to generation within each culture.

AUTHOR'S PREFACE

The line that separates drug use from drug abuse differs from culture to culture and from person to person within each culture. A parent in France might be horrified to see his or her child use a hallucinogenic drug such as LSD, but an Indian father in the South American jungle would watch proudly as his son endures a rite of passage involving the use of psychoactive plants. An American parent might be alarmed to see his or her child smoking a marijuana cigarette, while at the same time that child might be dismayed to see a parent behaving badly after having had too much to drink at a party.

The perception of what constitutes drug abuse in a particular culture or even among a particular generation depends on customs as well as laws. This in no way implies, however, that it is safe to use a drug for any other than its intended medical use (if any), regardless of whether or not it is used in a traditional cultural context. Nor does it excuse the drug addict or overlook the tragic toll of deaths related to drug overdose. It does, however, require that any discussion of what constitutes drug abuse take into account social norms and traditions, as well as the effect the presumed abuse has on the society as a whole.

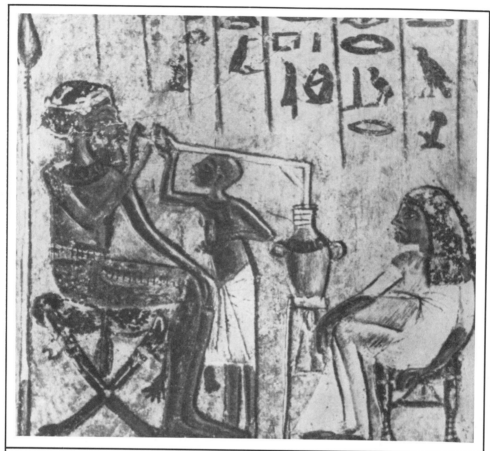

An ancient Egyptian wall painting of a man drinking beer. Drug abuse has existed since ancient times; some people have always had the desire to transcend ordinary consciousness through artificial means.

Drugs of Choice

Just as abuse varies from culture to culture, so do the drugs of abuse. The choice of drugs abused in a society depends mainly on the life-style and needs of the user, the availability and cost of the drugs, and peer pressure. Similarly, the experience desired or the effects that are sought often vary from user to user. The swaggering young Australian blue-collar workers who enjoy raucous drinking bouts in the "bloodhouse" bars of their country seek an experience that is vastly different from that desired by the Polynesian priests and chieftains who gather for the ceremonial consumption of kava, an intoxicating beverage. And the ambitious young English stockbroker who snorts cocaine to give him the burst of energy and confidence he thinks he needs to beat the competition is looking for a different effect than the one sought by a despondent, unemployed inner-city resident in America who uses heroin to forget his problems.

Still other drug users are just looking for "kicks." These people, willing to try anything at least once, often become polydrug users, possibly using one to get them high and another to level them out after they crash from the first. It is this desire to try anything once that may lead curious youths to sniff the toxic fumes of solvents such as model airplane glue or cause people to experiment with treacherous "designer drugs" concocted in homemade labs and sold on the street.

The Root of the Drug Abuse Problem

The root of the drug abuse problem is an ancient one. It is the desire, demonstrated by human beings since the very beginnings of time, to transcend ordinary consciousness through artificial means. Whether to heighten the joys of living, escape the woes of depression, or explore the mysteries of the mind, drug use and abuse have existed in almost every culture throughout the world.

In this volume we will explore the traditions that surround drug use in different cultures and the trends in modern societies that have led to a drug problem of epidemic proportions. We will consider the varied history of drug use first by region, and then by drug within the region. We will begin with alcohol, perhaps the oldest and most widely abused drug, and then go on to consider other substances of abuse, including marijuana, heroin, cocaine, hallucinogens, and tranquilizers. As we will see, it turns out that the horrors, contradictions, and complications of drug use and abuse around the world are born of the horrors, contradictions, and complications of the cultures of the world.

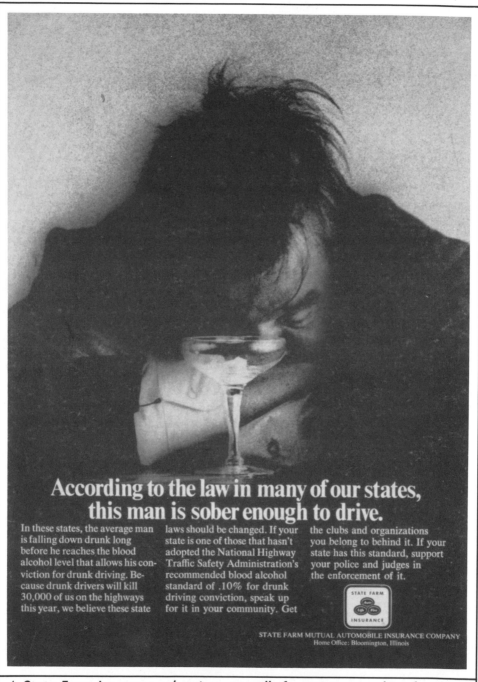

According to the law in many of our states, this man is sober enough to drive.

In these states, the average man is falling down drunk long before he reaches the blood alcohol level that allows his conviction for drunk driving. Because drunk drivers will kill 30,000 of us on the highways this year, we believe these state laws should be changed. If your state is one of those that hasn't adopted the National Highway Traffic Safety Administration's recommended blood alcohol standard of .10% for drunk driving conviction, speak up for it in your community. Get the clubs and organizations you belong to behind it. If your state has this standard, support your police and judges in the enforcement of it.

STATE FARM INSURANCE

STATE FARM MUTUAL AUTOMOBILE INSURANCE COMPANY
Home Office: Bloomington, Illinois

A State Farm Insurance advertisement calls for stricter penalties for drunk drivers. Although alcohol use pervades American society, knowledge of its dangers is also becoming more widespread.

CHAPTER 1

ALCOHOL USE AND ABUSE IN NORTH AMERICA

As a young woman stepped off the curb to cross a New York City street at about 3:00 A.M. on the morning of October 19, 1986, a car driven by a 26-year-old investment banker suddenly bore down on her. The car slammed into the woman, a 17-year-old student-body president of a Manhattan high school. The driver, drunk at the wheel, sped on, leaving the young woman lying in the street.

The following year a judge of the state supreme court sentenced the drunk driver to two and two-thirds to eight years in state prison. "You have caused the death of an exceptional person, one whose life showed great promise," the judge told the driver, before ordering him to be jailed immediately.

The same year Dr. Lawrence S. Harris, a North Carolina state medical examiner, reported at a national medical meeting the results of a survey of another kind of tragic accident — one that occurs routinely in a much different part of the country: the poor, rural areas of the South and Southwest.

Dr. Harris said that about every two weeks a drunk pedestrian wandering along a dark stretch of country road seeks relief from the bite of the chilly night air by lying down on the pavement, which retains the heat from the day. Over the course of 5 years ending in 1984, cars ran over and killed 136 people who were lying in the road at night. Tennessee counted 31 of these so-called lying-in-the-road deaths from 1980 through 1984, and Georgia officials tallied 21 from 1984 to 1986.

The culture of the young female pedestrian who became the victim of a drunk driver in New York City is a world away from the life-style of the poor, rural alcohol abuser who exposes himself to the dangers of a dark country road. The tragic consequences of alcohol abuse, however, were the same.

In the United States, the widespread availability and popularity of alcohol has helped to insinuate this drug into all levels of society, affecting virtually all racial, political, economic, and age groups. Most people now realize that the corporate businessman, the white-collar worker, the Hollywood actor, the journalist, the physician, and the next-door neighbor are as likely to be alcoholics as the stereotypical skid row bum.

The Plight of the American Indians

Although no one group is immune to the lure of alcoholism, there are several that appear to be especially susceptible, or that require special consideration. Among these are the American Indians.

On February 23, 1945, during the ferocious fighting in the Pacific theater of World War II, Ira Hayes, a Pima Indian from the Gila Indian Reservation in Phoenix, Arizona, helped four of his fellow Marines and a Navy corpsman hoist an American flag atop Mount Suribachi, on the island of Iwo Jima. A journalist snapped a picture of the event. On Veterans Day 1954, Ira Hayes and two other survivors of that memorable moment stood in Arlington, Virginia, and watched as officials unveiled a 75-foot-tall bronze statue modeled after that photograph.

Two months later, Hayes was found dead by the side of the road on the Indian reservation near Sacaton, Arizona.

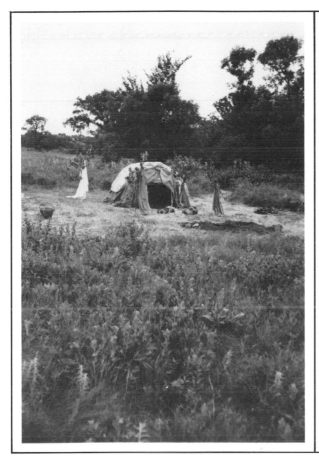

A Sioux Indian sweat lodge. These saunalike structures, originally used in healing ceremonies, are also sometimes used as a treatment for alcoholism among American Indians.

Medical officials cited alcoholism and freezing weather conditions as factors in his death.

Deprived of the open land that supported them for centuries and relegated to reservations located on unfertile land, many Indians have lived for years in poverty, despair, and neglect. Pride in their heritage too often has given way to a poor self-image, especially among the young, who probably felt the brunt of the discrimination directed at the American Indians. The ready availability of alcohol made this drug an ideal escape from the pain and prejudice of everyday life.

Often, their poverty drives American Indians to consume nonbeverage alcohol (NBA), such as hair spray and spray disinfectants. A 1987 report in the *Journal of Studies on Alcohol* pointed out that abuse of "Montana Gin," which is hair spray or spray disinfectant mixed with juice or soda, occurs in at least 14 states.

According to a 1985 Indian Health Service report, death from alcoholism among Indians and Eskimos between the ages of 25 and 34 was 11.2 times higher than for non-Indians of the same age group. Among 35- to 44-year-olds, it was 7.7 times higher, and among 45- to 54-year olds, 4.8 times higher.

Furthermore, according to 1983 statistics from the Department of Health and Human Services, there were 28.9 alcohol-related deaths among each 100,000 American Indians, compared with 6.1 deaths per 100,000 for all other ethnic groups.

In response to the growing problem of alcohol abuse among American Indians, those Indians living on reservations in many areas across the United States began to incorporate the Indian tradition of the healing sweat lodge into their alcoholism-treatment programs.

The healing sweat lodge was used by several tribes for religious purification and medical treatment. Though originally constructed of ash or willow saplings covered by buffalo skins, the modern version is usually constructed with blankets or canvas. The person in need of treatment must sit in the lodge while water is poured over stones that have been heated in a fire. This is done repeatedly over a period of time, producing large amounts of steam similar to a sauna effect. The participants sweat profusely during this body-cleansing ritual.

An even more ancient practice was brought to the Pine Ridge Indian Reservation in South Dakota in 1986 by medical experts from New York City. The *Rapid City Journal* of South Dakota reported that the team had trained counselors on the staff of Project Recovery, an alcoholism prevention and referral program on the reservation, in the technique and use of acupuncture, an ancient Chinese therapeutic technique. The counselors inserted 4 or 5 needles into each ear of a patient for up to 45 minutes. The treatment, which was effective for up to 72 hours, eased withdrawal symptoms and craving for alcohol.

In addition, Estele Fielder, a 46-year-old former alcoholic who grew up on the Cheyenne River Sioux Indian Reservation in South Dakota, began a group called American Indians for Sobriety in 1987. The organization was conceived as a network of recovered alcoholics that would provide role models for American Indian children on and off reservations, thus attempting to reverse the current trend for many of these young people to become alcohol abusers.

Blacks, Alcohol, and Advertising

In 1987, the Center for Science in the Public Interest voiced concern about alcohol abuse among blacks. In a report titled "Marketing Booze to Blacks," the center criticized what it described as the alcoholic beverage industry's strategy of saturating the black community with advertising that extols the joys of drinking.

Although they have been discriminated against for centuries in education, politics, business, and access to the media, in the 20th century blacks have emerged as an economic and thus consumer force to be reckoned with. In response, various industries have targeted them for aggressive advertising. Among these are the cigarette and alcoholic beverage industries.

The center's report on advertising in black communities pointed out that a higher proportion of the alcohol industry's advertising is placed in magazines and on radio stations with predominantly black rather than white audiences. In addition, the alcohol industry visibly supports black sports and civic events.

Although a higher proportion of whites than blacks use alcohol, the negative impact of drinking falls disproportionately on blacks, according to the report. This is due to the promotion of higher-alcohol beverages such as malt liquor and fortified wines and the fact that many blacks have less health care—especially preventive care—available to them.

Citing data from the National Institutes of Health, the report states that cirrhosis of the liver, a disease that is frequently associated with alcohol abuse, is twice as common among blacks as among whites. Moreover, a study published in the *Journal of Studies on Alcohol* in 1986 identified a tendency among inner-city blacks to drink and then encourage their spouse or living companion to drink with them. Under such conditions, there is a lack of support for sobriety.

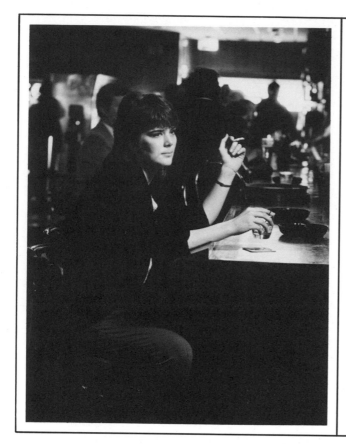

The drinking patterns of male and female alcoholics vary. Men with drinking problems tend to drink with large groups of friends, whereas similarly afflicted women usually drink alone.

The Female Alcoholic

In the past, when most people thought of alcoholism, they thought of it as a problem associated with men. In more recent years, however, the medical community has come to recognize that many women suffer from the disease of alcoholism. In light of this discovery, newly developed programs have begun to address the special needs of the female alcoholic.

One such organization is Women for Sobriety, Inc. (WFS), founded in 1976 by two-time Alcoholics Anonymous (AA) dropout Jean Kirkpatrick. Kirkpatrick started the organization after discovering that the AA rate for recovery was significantly higher for men than for women. With this in mind, she set out to create a program that dealt specifically with the needs of female alcoholics.

Kirkpatrick points out that many housewives enjoy "an alcoholic's paradise" because they are alone for a large part of each day and have time for binge drinking. But even those women who have taken up jobs and careers outside the home can be vulnerable to alcohol abuse, succumbing to the pressures and demands of the workplace.

Other factors that contribute to the problems unique to female alcoholics, according to Kirkpatrick, are the cultural differences between men and women, which are often reflected in their drinking patterns. Whereas men most often drink in public, with large groups of friends, women tend to drink privately, at home, with a single companion or alone.

Once they have admitted their problem with alcohol and attempt to control it, men usually receive peer support, especially in the workplace, where they are likely to remain employed. Women, on the other hand, are often ostracized for being alcoholics and more often than not are dismissed from their jobs. It is also interesting, if somewhat sad, to note that whereas 9 out of 10 wives elect to remain with a husband recovering from alcohol abuse, only 1 in 10 husbands is willing to do the same.

In 1987, the *Wall Street Journal* reported that women bought 17 percent of the beer sold in the United States, a figure that translates into $6.5 billion in sales. The article explained that many women were attracted to beer after the introduction of light, lower-calorie beers in the 1970s.

Moreover, the Centers for Disease Control reported in 1987 that even though more men than women drink heavily (two or more drinks of beer, wine, or liquor every day), women appear to have less resistance to illness caused by alcohol.

Children: The Youngest Victims

Among those who suffer the most and perhaps the most senselessly from the effects of alcoholism are children. In 1987, according to the National Institute on Alcohol Abuse and Alcoholism, it was estimated that more than 28 million Americans were children of alcoholics. Many of these children grow up with a fear of marriage or parenthood or become overly devoted to a spouse addicted to drugs, gambling, or some other self-destructive substance or activity.

Although many of these children of alcoholics may have been physically or sexually abused by an alcoholic parent, a large number themselves become alcoholics or drug abusers. In fact, children of alcoholics are four times more likely than other children to become alcoholics, according to studies done by Dr. Marc A. Schuckit, a psychiatrist at the University of California at San Diego.

In response to this problem, groups such as Alateen and Children of Alcoholics have instituted programs to reach out to young children still living with alcoholics and to adults who were the children of alcoholics.

Thousands of teens each year die on this nation's streets and highways from the deadly combination of drinking and driving, and alcohol abuse is associated with about half of the 44,000 deaths that occur on American highways each year. It is this problem that led Robert Anastas, a high school coach and guidance counselor, to found Students Against Driving Drunk (SADD), an educational, peer-group organization.

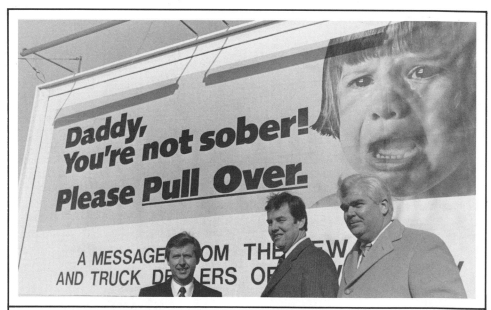

New Jersey governor Thomas Kean (center) with officials of the state automobile dealers' association in front of an anti-drunk driving poster. A parent's drinking problem can traumatize his or her entire family.

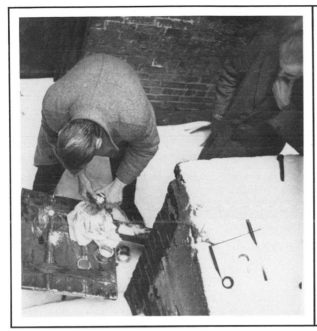

A rare photo of a street person making "squeeze," a cloudy pink nonbeverage alcohol (NBA). This potentially lethal concoction is made by heating Sterno and then pushing it through a rag to obtain alcohol. The mixture is cooled down with water before it is consumed.

According to a 1987 report by the Centers for Disease Control, males aged 18 to 34 show the highest incidence of drinking and driving. It is this group that benefits the most from SADD, which educates teens to refuse to drink and drive despite pressure from friends. SADD has even created a parent-teen contract allowing a teen who has been drinking or is with a driver who has been drinking to call his or her parents for a ride home at night. The parents agree not to discuss the incident until the next day. Thus far, SADD has been highly praised for this "safe ride" measure, which has proven quite effective. And Mothers Against Drunk Driving (MADD) has also helped to force states to treat drunk drivers harshly. Unfortunately, some drunk drivers have begun to ride bicycles. As a result, the number of drunk bicyclists killed in accidents around the United States is on the rise.

Drink of Desperation: Nonbeverage Alcohol

On Franklin Avenue in Minneapolis, Minnesota, police noticed that street people were mixing Lysol disinfectant, which contains ethyl alcohol, with water, juice, or soda. The "Franklin Avenue Cocktail," as it was called, left its mark on that section of the city in the form of dozens of empty disinfectant cans littering the street.

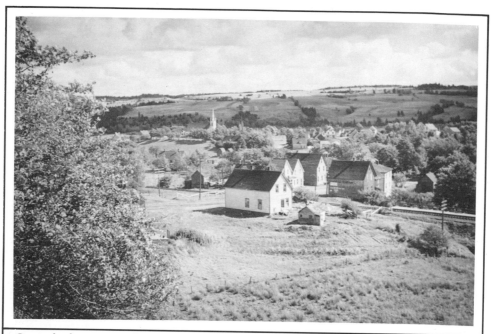

Canada has a number of small communities that boast few entertainment options. The only social life in many of these relatively isolated towns centers around the neighborhood pub.

Consumption of nonbeverage alcohol (NBA) is not unusual, according to a 1985 report in the *Journal of Studies on Alcohol*. For example, 15 to 20% of alcoholics hospitalized in Veterans Administration alcoholism-treatment units report having used NBA drinks at least once. And an informal survey in a private community hospital concluded that 6 to 10% of affluent alcoholics also use NBAs.

Many alcoholics use NBA on a regular basis, often consuming large quantities of such alcohol-containing substances as mouthwash, aftershave lotion, hair tonic, rubbing alcohol, and canned cooking fuel. These items are sold in stores that are usually open at times that liquor stores are closed.

Consumers of NBA often cite the ready availability of the product they drink, rather than the cheaper cost, as the reason they use it. Indeed, NBA use is prevalent in prisons, hospitals, and other places where access to beverage alcohol is limited or impossible.

The Long History of Drinking in Canada

During the 18th century, after French and British immigrants brought rum and brandy to what is now Canada, the native Indians and Eskimos became heavy users of alcohol. Accounts of social occasions during this time indicate widespread use and abuse of alcohol, followed often by "noisy, riotous, drunken meetings often terminating in violent quarrels and sometimes even in bloodshed," according to one 19th-century commentator.

In response to the mayhem, a temperance movement supported mostly by Methodist, Presbyterian, and Baptist churches became active during the early 1900s. Today, Canada has close government control of all aspects of the manufacture, distribution, and sale of alcohol. Yet according to a historical account published in 1985 in the *British Journal of Addiction*, " ... popular support for drunkenness still remains in Canada; national and local cultural events, for example, New Year's Eve ... and indeed most spectator sports, often involve heavy drinking."

The account points out that, as in Scandinavian countries, "there is an excellent support for alcohol research which flows out of a long preoccupation with drinking as a social problem." Unfortunately, there is also a scarcity of data available on the problem.

A more recent report in the same journal pointed out that 78% of adult Canadians use alcohol. In the numerous smaller communities of this vast country, where there are relatively few entertainment options, some people become regulars at a particular public drinking place. As in the United States, unmarried men and women commonly frequent a favorite bar or nightclub. And in Canada, as in the United States, drunk driving remains a serious problem.

The problems associated with alcohol and alcoholism in Canada were summarized for *Macleans* magazine in 1986 by Alan Podsadowski, director of the Alternative Substance Abuse Treatment Program in North Vancouver: "Alcohol will always be the number one problem. There is no question that if anyone tried to market alcohol today for the first time, it would never pass." This is as true for the United States as it is in Canada, and probably throughout the world.

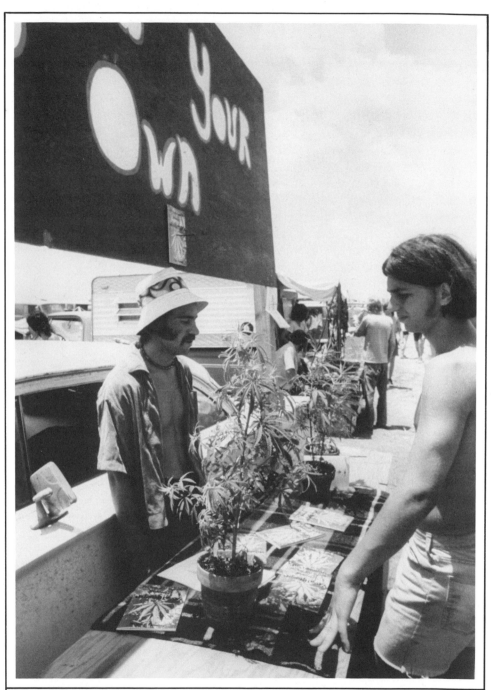

A 1971 photograph shows a man selling books on how to grow marijuana plants. In the late 1960s and early 1970s, marijuana became the drug of choice among self-styled young American rebels.

CHAPTER 2

DRUG ABUSE IN NORTH AMERICA

A 1985 survey conducted by the National Institute on Drug Abuse (NIDA) disclosed that at least 37 million Americans —about 1 out of 5 people 12 years or older—admitted having used one or more illicit drugs in the previous year. More than 10% had used an illicit drug at least once in the past month.

Marijuana Use in the United States and Canada

During the early part of the 20th century, marijuana was the drug of choice among jazz musicians and bohemians. During the late 1960s and early 1970s, however, the drug entered the mainstream, as American youth en masse embraced it as a badge of rebellion against establishment values and traditions. The self-styled rebels and nonconformists of this era became the parents of the 1980s, with young children or teenagers of their own.

A *Providence Journal* report entitled "Marijuana: Growing Up in Smoke" illustrated this development. The newspaper described how a young girl, now in the care of a guardian, "still waves to the drug dealers assembled around a fountain . . . as she rides by in her guardian's car. She remembers them from the days when she was just 7 or 8 and her mother would give her money to go down to the fountain and pick up some marijuana."

Marijuana smoking is now firmly entrenched in American society. Office workers, construction workers, and medical professionals are among the millions of regular users of this drug.

Despite the widespread acceptance of marijuana smoking, the NIDA Household Survey found that the number of marijuana users actually declined from 20 million to 18.2 million between 1982 and 1985. But of those, 6 million people said they were regular users. And 1 in 6 Americans 20 to 40 years old said they smoked marijuana at least once a month. About 24% of youths have used marijuana at some time during their lives. In addition, at least one out of every 25 high school seniors smokes marijuana on a daily basis.

In recent years, health officials have grown particularly concerned about the effects of long-term, regular use of marijuana on intellectual performance and memory. Some officials also fear that marijuana is a "gateway" drug; that is, one that serves as an important step toward later abuse of other drugs, especially cocaine.

In Canada, marijuana possession remains illegal and the streamlining of arrest and arraignment procedures in the criminal justice system has helped to thwart efforts at decriminalization. Indeed, since 1974, at least 25,000 persons have been arrested each year for possessing cannabis (the plant from which marijuana and hashish is derived) each year.

A recent study of cannabis users showed that most "cannabis criminals" were young, single males who used the drug at least twice a week. In 1981, those males were more likely than their peers in 1974 to be unemployed and living at home with parents — probably because of the general decline in economic prospects for young Canadians during that period.

Cocaine History Repeats Itself

A cocaine epidemic gripped the United States from about 1885 until the 1920s. Sparked by the legal sale of cocaine in drugstores and through the mail, the drug's presence in a variety of soft drinks, and the general belief that the drug was safe, nonaddictive, and beneficial, cocaine use spread rapidly.

After the first few years of euphoric use, however, Americans became increasingly alarmed at the destructive poten-

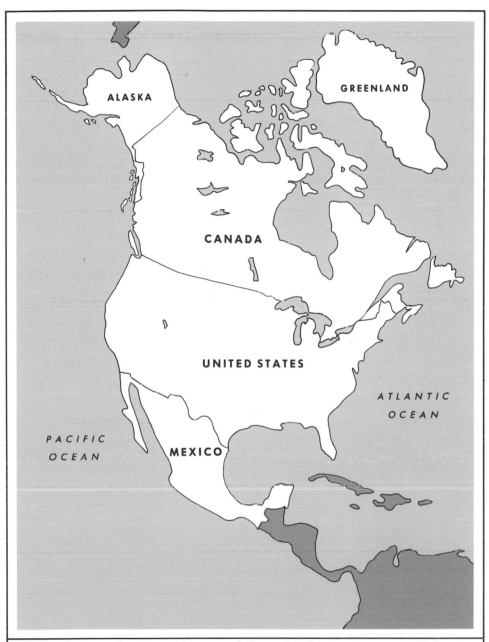

North America. *A sophisticated drug distribution system trafficks a variety of drugs from Latin America, the Middle East, and Asia into Canada and the United States.*

tial of cocaine. Many Americans began to associate the drug with addiction, paranoia, and crime. Thereafter, society as a whole rejected the drug, and cocaine use declined substantially.

Forgetting the lessons of the first epidemic, Americans began using cocaine again during the 1970s. The strict laws that had been passed to control cocaine abuse so many years before seemed unnecessary; many people now thought that cocaine was reasonably safe and relatively nonaddictive. It became the "champagne of drugs," and acquired a glamorous image. Originally cocaine was the drug of pimps, prostitutes, and other shadowy figures on the edge of society. But its use soon spread to actors, models, athletes, artists, jazz musicians, designers, and business professionals.

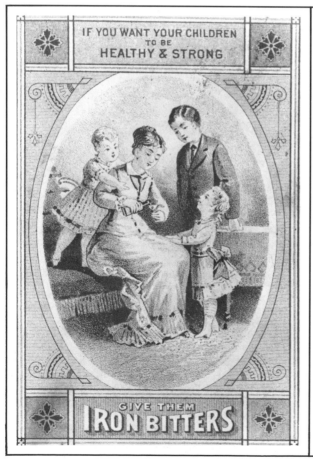

During the late 19th and early 20th centuries, cocaine was an ingredient in a variety of over-the-counter elixirs, such as Iron Bitters.

IF YOU WANT YOUR CHILDREN TO BE HEALTHY & STRONG

GIVE THEM IRON BITTERS

Although the number of people who used cocaine regularly (that is, at least once during the past 30 days), grew from 1.6 million in 1977 to 5.8 million in 1985, according to NIDA statistics, the current trend seems to be away from cocaine use. A January 1988 article in the *New York Times* reported that cocaine use among high school seniors had dropped for the first time in 13 years. This report, based on a survey done by the University of Michigan's Institute for Social Research, raised the hope that the battle may be turning in the war against cocaine.

Despite the decrease in the number of cocaine users, a new problem looms on the horizon. Crack, a cheap, smokable form of cocaine, has found its way onto the streets and playgrounds of many major U.S. cities. And, unfortunately, crack use has not followed the overall trend of declining drug abuse.

Although the drug has found some users among affluent young people, crack has taken its greatest toll among the despairing, uneducated poor of the inner city. There, the need to obtain money to buy crack has bred crime, destroying neighborhoods, creating empty stores and vacant lots, and frightening residents.

By the mid-1980s, the press was reporting countless lurid stories of how addiction to cocaine — especially crack — led respectable people to theft, prostitution, and murder to get money for the drug. In response, religious and lay organizations across the country began campaigning against these drugs in an effort to save their neighborhoods.

Narcotic Abuse Takes a Dangerous Turn

The crack epidemic in the United States threatened to shift public attention away from the problem of heroin addiction. But like the cocaine problem, which became a crack epidemic, heroin addiction in the United States also took a dangerous turn in the 1980s, and landed back on the front page of newspapers around the world.

Acquired Immune Deficiency Syndrome (AIDS), a deadly, incurable, viral disease that ravages the immune system, found easy access to a large pool of victims: intravenous drug users who shared needles with drug addicts already carrying the virus.

Tragically, even AIDS has not stopped the steady abuse of heroin. Addicts still seek out drug dealers, and some dealers on the street have begun to lure addicts by hawking their wares as package deals combining heroin and used needles that are sold as new needles. "Get the good needles, don't get the bad AIDS," called out one dealer observed by health professionals studying the street scene in New York City. In early 1988, Governor Cuomo decided to permit New York City to provide clean needles to hundreds of addicts to prevent the spread of AIDS.

Experts warn that drug addicts are an important potential bridge that may allow AIDS to enter the general population through heterosexual contact with nonaddicts. But the exact number of heroin users is difficult to calculate because addicts are usually hidden from the public eye. Often they are criminals or others living on the edge of society, although some secretive middle- and upper-class citizens are also part of the addict population. Various analytical models over the years have put the number of heroin addicts in the United States at between 400,000 and 600,000, about 200,000 of whom are in New York City.

Heroin has consistently been used by less than one-half of one percent of the population since the early 1970s, according to NIDA figures. In recent years, the addict population has remained fairly stable. As the population of those initiated into heroin abuse between the mid-1960s and mid-1970s aged, however, there was an increase in the number of those abusers either requiring emergency room treatment or dying.

Heroin may yet stage a vicious comeback now that a "black tar" version of the drug has become popular among certain segments of society. Cheap, pure, and deadly, black tar heroin is a new form of Mexican heroin that began inundating many U.S. cities during the 1980s.

Farmers in the northern Mexican states of Durango, Sinaloa, and Sonora use a simple procedure to produce a form of heroin that is either sticky, like roofing tar, or hard, like coal. As much as 45 times purer than conventional Mexican heroin, it has increased the danger of overdose among unsuspecting—or desperate—users.

According to a U.S. Drug Enforcement Administration report, black tar heroin is available in all established Mexican-American communities in the United States. The drug is smuggled in, primarily by illegal aliens and migrant workers.

CHAPTER 3

ALCOHOL USE AND ABUSE IN EUROPE

In the winter of 1980, strong gales churned the sea around the rugged shorelines of the Connemara Islands, off the western coast of Ireland. Moonshiners in small, sturdy boats slipped across the waters unmolested by the Irish police, who had to call off their forays against the smugglers because their own inflatable boats could not weather the turbulent waters.

On the mainland, the Irish pubs were trying to weather a decrease in business. More than half of that nation's pubs failed to make a profit that year. High bar taxes and hard economic times had quenched the thirst of many pub regulars. Despite the important role pubs have traditionally played in the social lives of the Irish, a depressing quiet settled over many of these establishments. Nevertheless, the pub tradition did not die out, especially among the young.

The Irish not only drink less than do people of several other countries (the United States, for example), but they also appear to drink for different reasons than do their counterparts. A comparative study of the drinking habits of Irish and American college students, published in 1987 in the *International Journal of the Addictions*, concluded that Irish females "look to alcohol to help them feel less restricted by social conventions, and. . . . those who drink most heavily do so to obtain greater sexual responsiveness."

Although the consumption of alcohol on a daily basis has traditionally been a part of many European societies, there is evidence of escalating alcohol abuse problems in many of these countries.

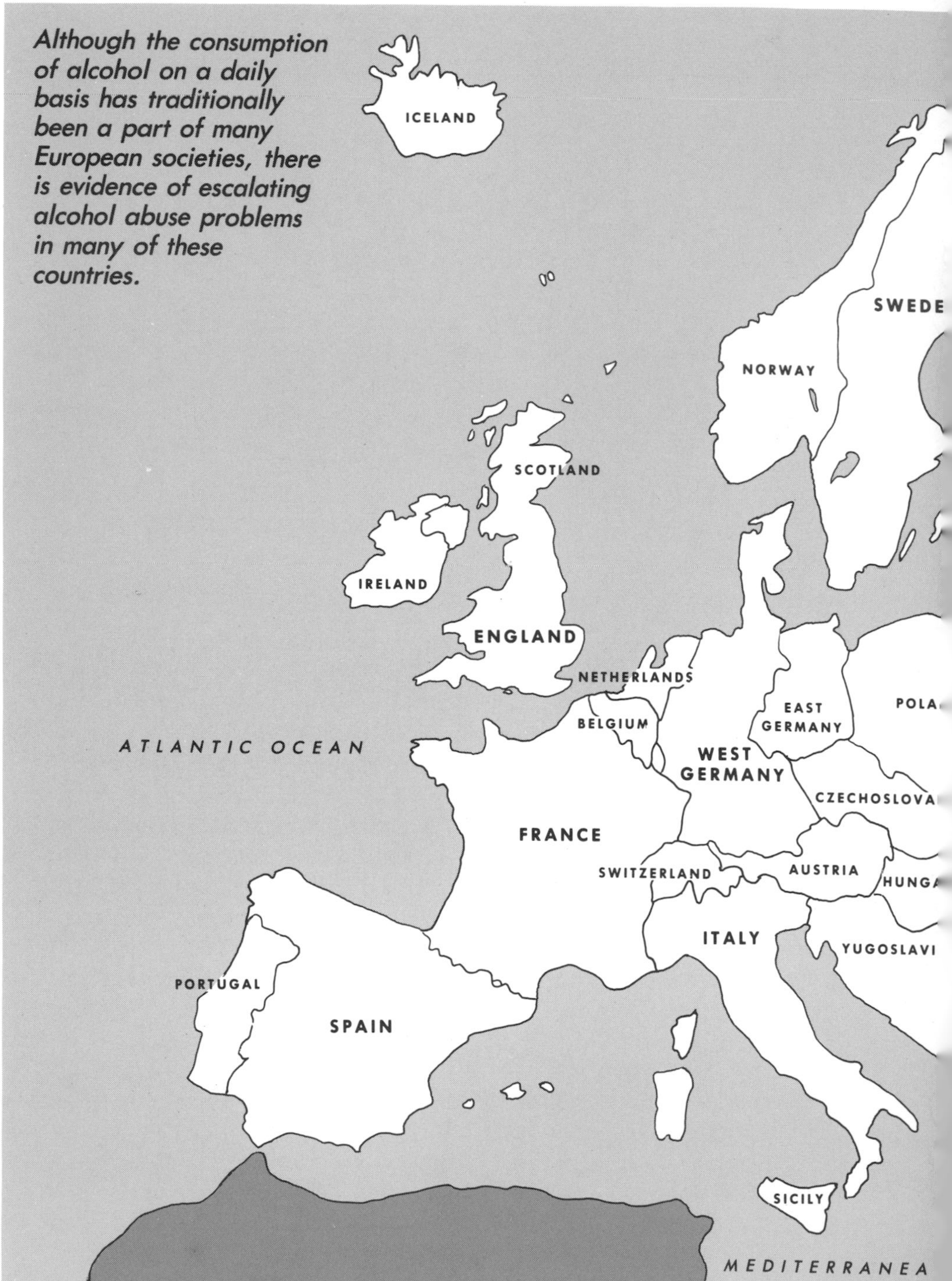

ICELAND

SWEDE

NORWAY

SCOTLAND

IRELAND

ENGLAND

NETHERLANDS

BELGIUM

EAST GERMANY

POLA

ATLANTIC OCEAN

WEST GERMANY

CZECHOSLOVA

FRANCE

SWITZERLAND

AUSTRIA

HUNGA

ITALY

YUGOSLAVI

PORTUGAL

SPAIN

SICILY

MEDITERRANEA

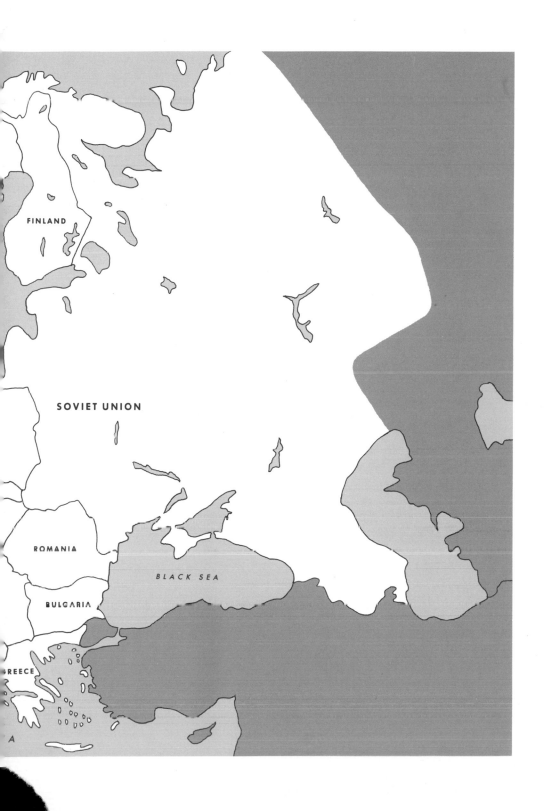

FINLAND

SOVIET UNION

ROMANIA

BLACK SEA

BULGARIA

GREECE

A

Significantly, Irish women face a more repressive society than do American women, because in Ireland contraception, divorce, and abortion are illegal. Furthermore, women have no legal rights or status in Ireland if they separate from their husbands. Apparently, then, some Irish women drink as a way to rebel against what they perceive as a repressive society.

The study also found that young Irish women are far less concerned about getting into trouble with the authorities as a result of their drinking. According to the study, this attitude is probably due to the "greater tolerance the Irish have toward drunken behavior.... and the tendency to view problems associated with 'the drink' with some amusement."

Rebelliousness seemed a part of the drinking attitudes of Irish men as well. "The Irish nation has traditionally been casual in its adherence to civil authority and laws," the report's author points out, "likely harking back to feelings about once being subjected to British rule...." The Irish men also tended to associate drinking with creativity and were less caught up in trying to maintain a success-oriented, "macho" image than their counterparts in the United States.

Although studies conducted in the United States have identified Irish Americans as a population at high risk for alcohol abuse problems, alcohol consumption in Ireland is no greater than in many other European countries. However, Ireland does appear to have a high rate of alcoholics among those who do drink.

Alcohol Use and Abuse in England

Alcohol has also played an important role in English history. Drinking was built into the very fabric of life as early as the 17th century. Socioeconomic factors virtually ensured heavy drinking. Beer was substituted for drinking water, which was often contaminated, and brewing and distilling used up grain surpluses. Physicians prescribed wine for a variety of ills. And in an age when the common people routinely faced pain, poverty, cold, hunger, and oppression, alcohol beckoned with the enticing promise of forgetfulness.

Today, beer is still the most popular drink in England, perhaps reflecting the long history of pubs. Although many of the health-conscious British now drink mineral water or low-alcohol beer with their meals, nearly 1 million Britons

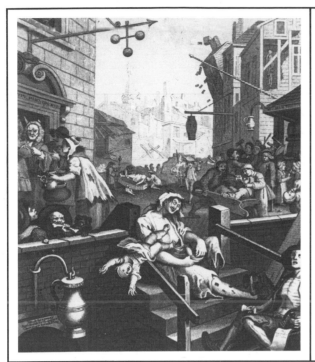

Beer Street and Gin Lane, by the 18th-century artist William Hogarth. By Hogarth's time the British were importing some 10 million gallons of Dutch gin annually, and public drunkenness was rampant in many urban areas.

still have a drinking problem, according to the *Economist* magazine. The magazine reports, though, that heavy drinking, like smoking, "is increasingly concentrated at the bottom of the social scale."

Nevertheless, it seems that English women of all social classes are now drinking more. These women often use pubs as a getaway from the drudgery of home life and a convenient place to gather with friends. But in small villages this is not always easy. For example, a study of the efforts of women in English villages to break into the social life of the male-dominated pubs found that most males generally did not find it acceptable for women to enter such establishments unaccompanied by men.

The study, published in the *Sociological Review*, documented the efforts of women (some of whom were married) to find acceptance by forming teams that competed in darts, a common pub sport. This activity legitimized their presence in pubs and helped them to gain acceptance among pub regulars.

In England, drinking is also increasing among young people. A survey by the Royal College of Psychiatrists found that a third of all 13-year-old English children drink alcohol on the average of once every other day. Furthermore, half of all automobile accidents involving teenagers are linked to alcohol.

The London *Times Educational Supplement* reported in 1987 that drunkenness among school-aged teens is "increasing alarmingly" and noted that abuse of alcohol may lead to abuse of other drugs. For the first time in this century, according to a report by the country's Department of Health and Social Security, 16 year olds are more at risk from drunkenness than people aged 20 to 60.

In 1986, Britain's Adam Smith Institute, an independent research organization, recommended that England follow Scotland's lead in reducing alcohol-related problems by relaxing licensing laws governing drinking establishments. In a report titled "Time to Call Time," the institute pointed out

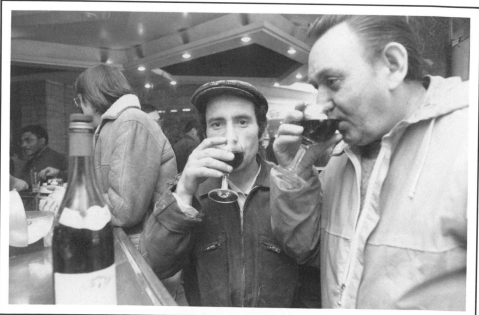

French workers enjoy a glass of wine during a break. France, one of the major wine-producing countries, has the largest alcohol consumption per person 15 years or older in Europe.

that, since 1976, when business hours were extended in Scotland's drinking establishments, the traditional "beat the clock" attitude of heavy consumption before closing has diminished considerably. Underage drinking and convictions for drunkenness have decreased as well.

Drinking on the Continent

Across the English Channel, alcohol abuse is also of great concern. According to Dr. Rudolf Mader, a physician at a drug rehabilitation institute in Vienna, Austria, about 2.5% of the population in central Europe are alcoholics. This same figure, he points out, was also mentioned in similar studies done in the late-19th century.

In a 1984 article in the journal *Impact of Science on Society*, Dr. Mader pointed out that, especially in countries where alcoholic products are of great economic importance and drinking habits are well established, alcoholism appears to be a particularly intractable problem.

For example, France, a major wine-producing country, has the largest alcohol consumption per person 15 years of age and older in Europe. By 1984, alcohol was causing about 30,000 deaths a year in France, whereas deaths from other drugs totaled only about 150, according to Dr. Claude Olievenstein, a physician and researcher at several psychiatric hospitals in Paris.

Spain, another important wine-producing country, also has a major alcoholism problem, according to a 1984 report in *Impact* by Ramon Mendoza, a Spanish government health official. Although wine was still the main alcoholic beverage in Spain, consumption of beer and hard liquor had risen enormously in the past several years.

Alcohol in Northern Europe

The widespread abuse of alcohol in southern Europe seems ironic, considering that southern Europeans have an ancient image of their northern counterparts as hard drinkers with a tendency to be violent when drunk. Indeed, a 1986 report by Norwegian researchers on drinking in Iceland, Finland, Sweden, and Norway points out that the old drinking traditions are especially strong in Iceland and Finland. The study, published in the *British Journal of Addiction*, found that drinkers in Iceland were more likely to suffer hangovers or other physical discomfort, and to have been more boisterous or quarrelsome when drunk, than drinkers in the other Scandinavian countries.

In Iceland, drinking takes place among family or close friends, in groups called "quasi-kin" that are important social units in this cold, desolate, and sparsely populated country. According to a 1985 report in *Anthropological Quarterly*, boisterous drunkenness is generally condoned only when it occurs outside these settings — for example, at public functions such as large weekend parties. The report also points out that drunkenness at public functions permits Icelanders to "mingle freely, knowing that these social contacts are impermanent and thus non-threatening to the all-important 'kin' and drinking group."

Drinkers in Finland, although less likely than Icelanders to become violent when drunk, are more likely to suffer societal disapproval. This may be due to stricter social control in Finland over certain forms of behavior associated with the use of alcohol — even though Finland has the highest per capita consumption among all four countries.

The drinking experience in Norway and Sweden has evolved along lines closer to those of southern Europe, and this shift is reflected in more moderate levels of drinking. Moderate drinking at meals is more common in Sweden, but much less so in Iceland. However, in Norway and Sweden, as in Finland, drunkenness is condemned more readily than in Iceland. In all Scandinavian countries, drinking and working tend to be kept separate.

In 1976, the Swedish Parliament abolished the sale of medium-strong beer (3.6% alcohol), and replaced it with a 2.8% beer. This switch, coupled with a steady increase in the price of alcoholic beverages from 1979 to 1984, a decrease in mean income, a ban on alcohol advertising, and a ban on the Saturday sale of alcohol at state-owned liquor shops (the only outlets for alcoholic beverages besides restaurants), drove down the consumption of alcohol in Sweden. This decrease has also been encouraged by many municipalities and organizations, such as the Swedish Medical Association.

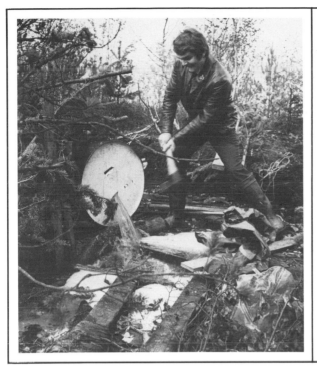

A Finnish policeman destroys an illegal still. Although Finland has the highest per capita alcohol consumption in Scandinavia, there is strict social control over drunken behavior.

According to a 1986 article in *Contemporary Drug Problems*, alcohol consumption in Greenland was curtailed through rationing in 1979. During this time consumers used coupon "points" that allowed them to buy alcoholic beverages. In response, thefts, burglaries, and muggings increased as criminals tried to obtain coupons, money to buy alcohol, or alcohol itself. A black market for coupons also developed, and alcohol smuggling increased, as did illegal home brewing of beer and distilling of hard liquor. At the same time, use of hashish rose significantly, and many people turned to non-beverage alcohol products such as glue and paint thinner.

Five weeks before the repeal of rationing in 1982, Greenland pulled out of the cooperative union of European countries called the European Economic Community or the Common Market. As a result, the country lost millions of dollars worth of grants from the Common Market. After the repeal of alcohol rationing later in 1982, however, alcohol consumption skyrocketed and millions of dollars in alcohol tax revenue poured into Greenland's treasury.

At the same time, it seemed as though rivers of beer were also pouring into Greenland, as Denmark's two main beer breweries, Carlsberg and Tuborg, worked three shifts around the clock in the summer of 1982 just to meet Greenland's demand. In June 1982, for example, Greenland, a country with an adult population of about 34,000, imported the equivalent of 6.7 million drinks, or 6.6 drinks per adult per day.

Beer Drinking Traditions in Germany

In German-speaking countries, too, there are old traditions of alcohol use. The production and consumption of wine dates back to the ancient Roman Empire. Today, according to the *British Journal of Addiction*, daily wine consumption is common in the Federal Republic of Germany's wine-producing regions. Elsewhere in that country, however, wine is more often drunk only on special occasions, partly because of its relatively high price.

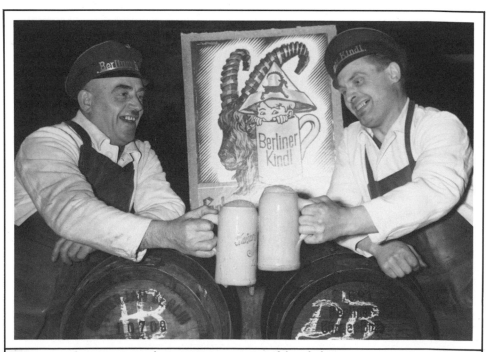

German brewery workers enjoy a stein of bock beer — an extra-strong beer with a 16% alcohol content. Three billion gallons of beer, West Germany's "national drink," are consumed in that nation each year.

Instead, the "national drink" of Germany is beer. With an annual consumption of 3 *billion* gallons (equivalent to 39 gallons for every man, woman, and child), the Federal Republic has the highest level of beer consumption in the world. The national drink is manufactured by large industrial breweries and hundreds of small brewers, according to centuries-old regulations that permit only the use of water, hops, malt, and yeast and bar the use of any additives.

Much of this beer is consumed by men who belong to their local *Stammtisch*, a subculture of beer-drinking fraternities. These fraternities, which exclude women, originated with the 19th-century trade guilds, whose members met over steins of beer to make deals and establish trade regulations. About 20% of German men belong to one of these fraternities, which now serve a mostly social function.

Hard liquor is also consumed regularly in West Germany, but mainly in the northern and eastern part of the country — and often with beer. There is a high level of alcohol abuse among German children, and there are about three times more alcohol-dependent men in the country than women.

Austria also has a history of heavy drinking, and today more than three-quarters of a million Austrians are problem drinkers, according to studies cited by Dr. Mader in his 1984 article in *Impact*. About 90% of those drinkers are men, mostly aged 35 to 50. According to Dr. Mader, skilled workers were most at risk among men for becoming alcohol abusers, followed by farmers, senior executives, and civil servants. There were no significant differences among women regarding the age or occupation most at risk.

Drinking: A Part of Russian History

Heavy drinking has been a tradition in the Soviet Union for centuries. The political and social upheavals during the 19th and early 20th centuries destabilized families and whole communities. According to a 1986 report on Soviet drinking patterns published in the *Annals of the New York Academy of Sciences*, this social upheaval, coupled with the fact that there was no history of effective prohibition or doctrine of moderation in drinking, contributed to a general abuse of alcohol.

The modern Soviet government, with its tight social and economic control over the population, has contributed to

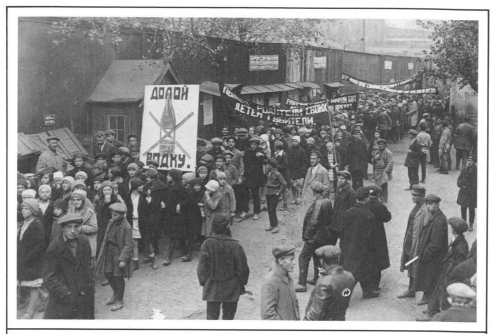

Soviet people protest the abuse of vodka during an antialcohol rally. It is estimated that alcohol abuse directly or indirectly claims from 300,000 to 500,000 Soviet lives a year.

the frustration of many of its citizens, whether intellectuals, artists, workers in inefficient state-run factories, or ordinary housewives who must spend hours in lines waiting to buy food at state-run stores. Alcohol abuse is one response to these everyday stresses, just as it is for the many people in Western countries who drink to forget their own problems.

There are groups in the Soviet Union, such as Muslims (who are strictly forbidden to drink alcohol) and Jews (whose religion fosters in them a respect for the wine they use in rituals and a contempt for drunkenness), that have cultural prohibitions against drug abuse that leave them relatively unscathed by the high rates of alcoholism. Other groups, however, have high rates of alcoholism. The blue-collar workers in the Slavic and Baltic regions, for example, have the highest rate of alcoholism in the country.

Reports published both inside and outside the Soviet Union have detailed the country's problems of increased rates of alcohol-related job absenteeism, birth defects, infant mortality, and child abuse. The drug has also been cited as being the leading cause of premature death.

The *Los Angeles Times* reported that alcohol abuse directly or indirectly claims about 300,000 to 500,000 Soviet lives a year, a rate 4 to 5 times that of the United States. Another sign of alcohol abuse in recent years was the appearance of newspaper reports in Moscow of high school students and teachers being disciplined for drunkenness.

In the 1980s, the Soviets began to take significant steps to curb the epidemic of alcoholism. The government doubled the cost of vodka and cut production levels of both vodka and wine. The legal drinking age was raised from 18 to 21, and alcohol was banned at official functions.

In response to these measures, between 1984 and 1987 consumption of state-produced vodka dropped from 8.4 liters per person to 4.4 liters, according to the *New York Times*. But that figure did not take into account Soviet consumption of *samogon*, a home-brewed liquor made mostly from sugar. In 1987, more than 100,000 Soviet citizens were hauled into court on moonshining charges, as the practice spread to all layers of society, including the intelligentsia. At the same time, there was a noticeable increase in the number of intoxicated people wandering the streets, as desperate drinkers turned to such NBAs as shaving lotion, insecticide, glue, shoe polish, and toxic industrial alcohol.

The sobriety campaign has had some positive effects, however. According to Interior Minister Aleksandr V. Vlasov, consumption was drastically cut, alcohol-related crime and road accidents have decreased, and the death rate from alcohol started falling for the first time in 20 years.

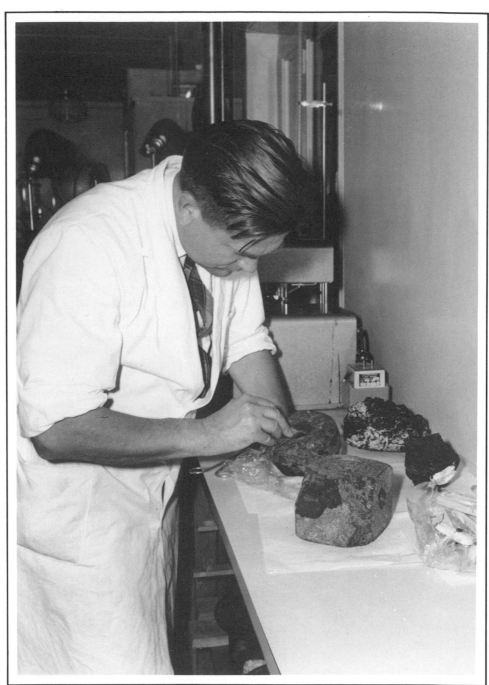

The United Nations Laboratory in Geneva, Switzerland, examines samples of illicit drugs seized by law-enforcement officials. These analyses seek to determine from which countries these samples come.

CHAPTER 4

DRUG ABUSE IN EUROPE

The use and abuse of marijuana is quite prevalent in Western Europe. Most of the marijuana that enters the Western European countries is smuggled in from the Near and Middle East, North Africa, countries south of the Sahara, and, increasingly, from South America.

A survey published in 1985 in the *British Journal of Addiction* found that in both England and Wales, men and women 25 to 34 years old who had completed their full-time education appeared to be the largest consumers of cannabis. This finding suggests that people who were students during the early 1970s, when use of the drug usually held great political and ideological significance abroad (as it did in the United States), were more likely than others to use the drug.

Marijuana is popular among many French adolescents as well, although the rate of use is much lower than it is in the United States. Like their peers in the United States, French youths often progress to marijuana use after first using beer or wine, then distilled spirits or cigarettes.

Marijuana

Amsterdam has tolerated drug use among young people for many years. During the 1960s, especially, youths from around the world flocked to this seaport city in the Netherlands to enjoy its relatively free-spirited attitude toward drug use. The government dropped criminal penalties against marijuana use in 1978, and by the 1980s, users were consuming marijuana cigarettes and cookies or "space cakes" baked with marijuana, which were on sale at any one of 200 "cannabis cafes." A service called Home Blow Couriers even offered free delivery of drugs on orders exceeding $12.50, according to a 1987 report in *Time* magazine.

Toleration of marijuana use in the Netherlands, however, has served to diffuse the drug's image as a form of rebellion against authority. Indeed, in 1984 the *Wall Street Journal* reported that fourth-fifths of the young people surveyed in the Netherlands said they had no interest in smoking marijuana. The government now believes that only 3% of the population are regular users. To a large extent, the image of the Netherlands as the "drug capital" of Europe has more to do with the activities of visitors than of the native population.

In Denmark, the Free State of Christiana serves as that country's drug capital. Eighty acres of homes, businesses, and woodlands established in 1971 as a self-proclaimed anarchist-hippie "nation," Christiana is an abandoned army base that is home to about 200 drug pushers who regard it "as one of Europe's great drug malls," according to a 1987 account in the *New York Times*. Dealers can often be found selling Moroccan hashish in the open-air market called Pusher Street.

Originally conceived as an experimental, free-living society unconstrained by authority of any sort, Christiana now suffers from pollution, racial violence, and overdevelopment. By the late 1980s, many residents began requesting regular police patrols, and the regional councils that oversee Christiana began to consider extending the ban on the sale of heroin and cocaine to hashish and marijuana — the so-called recreational drugs that supposedly epitomized the society's original live-and-let-live attitude.

The population of the Central Asian region of the Soviet Union has traditionally grown and used marijuana. Since the Soviet Union's strict anti-alcohol laws went into effect in

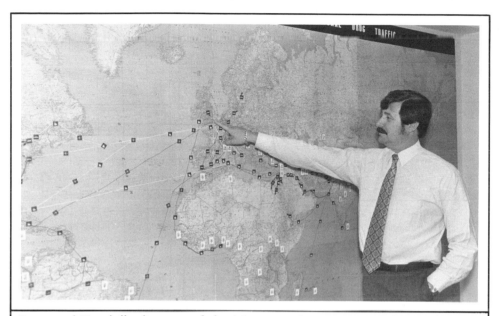

Raymond Kendall, director of the Narcotics Department at Interpol, points to Amsterdam, the Dutch city whose lenient policies regarding drug use attracted many young people in the 1960s and 1970s.

1985, however, consumption of marijuana in this area appears to have increased dramatically, according to a 1986 report in the Baltimore *Sun*. In Moscow, the increase in vodka prices and the closing of many liquor stores have led to long lines at open stores and an increase in the amount of hashish available. Moscow teenagers commonly talk about smoking *plan*, or marijuana. In response, the Soviet Union has stepped up its antidrug activities, including destroying crops and increasing the penalties for drug use.

Cocaine

During the 1980s, drug dealers, faced with a nearly saturated U.S. market for cocaine, established trafficking pipelines to Europe. As supplies increased and the price dropped, cocaine abuse spread rapidly throughout Europe from the wealthy to young people at almost all levels of society.

Much of Europe's cocaine supply comes from South America by way of Spain. By 1986, according to the *Christian Science Monitor*, Spain itself, awash in cocaine, was home to between 60,000 and 80,000 abusers of the drug and the number was increasing.

The problem is especially acute in France, the Federal Republic of Germany, and England. In France, where drug abusers were once considered only sick people, officials started an all-out campaign against drug addiction in 1986. The aim was to force people addicted to any illegal drug to undergo a cure or face imprisonment. As part of their new campaign, French officials sought to increase the number of hospital beds for addicts and to educate children about the dangers of drugs.

In England, London police set up telephone hot lines to gather information on the growing drug abuse problem among the young bankers and stockbrokers who dominate Britain's financial world. A survey done by the *Sunday Times* in 1987 found that 20% of the beds in Britain's leading private drug-treatment clinics were occupied by employees of some of Britain's biggest financial institutions. Experts blamed the stressful environment of the stock market for driving many people to cocaine abuse. Dr. Malcolm Carruthers, a specialist in treating stress in the workplace, said that the combination of stress and the opportunity to get rich puts pressure on people and "leads to the three-D syndrome — drink, drugs, and divorce."

In Eastern Europe and the Soviet Union, cocaine abuse is not prevalent. This is probably because of tighter border controls and stricter watch over chemicals and equipment — measures that discourage the importation and processing of cocaine.

The Heroin Problem Gets Complicated

In 1986, the daughter of a wealthy British politician died from an overdose of heroin. This highly publicized tragedy drew attention in England to the problem of drug abuse among the young, wealthy, privileged children of high society families in the United Kingdom and Europe. The young woman's death highlighted the immense problem of heroin abuse throughout Western Europe, where many thousands of citizens, both rich and poor, had succumbed to the drug. Heroin is widely available in Western Europe, and total quantities seized by authorities have increased yearly since 1984. The largest seizures have been made in the United Kingdom, the Netherlands, and France.

The Netherlands is home to an estimated 16,000 heroin addicts, a higher proportion of the population than in West Germany, Britain, or France. During the 1970s, Amsterdam licensed four cafes to distribute the drug to addicts. Following an increase in drug-related crime and 30 heroin-overdose deaths per year, the city ended the practice in 1980. Nevertheless, in 1987, heroin addicts were still routinely receiving advice and free methadone (a less dangerous heroin substitute) from a city medical bus "that comes quietly around each day like a milk wagon," according to an account in the *New York Times*.

To a great extent, drug abuse in the Netherlands reflects the activities of visitors and immigrants to that country rather than an indigenous problem. In addition to being an endpoint for much smuggled heroin, in the 1970s the Netherlands became a magnet for drug abusers — especially addicts from Germany — who took advantage of the ready supply of drugs and relatively tolerant attitude of the government toward

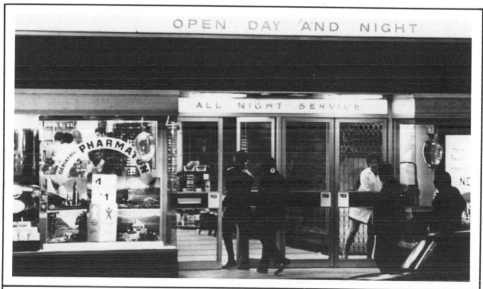

In England during the 1960s and early 1970s, heroin was available to addicts by prescriptions filled at ordinary drug stores. Unfortunately, much of the prescribed heroin found its way to the black market.

drugs. Of the 60 deaths related to hard drugs in that country in 1986, 35 were among visiting Germans, but only 16 were Dutch.

When Amsterdam police reported a steady rise in arrests for trafficking in hard drugs and in the amount of heroin seized, the country tripled the sentence for heroin trafficking to 12 years, with little chance for parole. Dutch authorities have also had to respond to the deadly threat of Acquired Immune Deficiency Syndrome (AIDS), which can be transmitted among intravenous drug addicts who share needles. In an effort to stem the spread of this disease, methadone buses began exchanging clean needles for used ones.

In 1986, England also decided to proceed with a pilot program of exchanging syringes in about a dozen treatment centers where drug addicts received counseling. Before 1968, Great Britain's illicit heroin market consisted almost entirely of legally prescribed, 100% pure heroin that was distributed to addicts under government supervision. According to the *British Journal of Addiction* (1985), however, addicts sold much of this heroin on the black market or exchanged it for goods or other drugs.

After 1968, the right to prescribe heroin and cocaine to addicts was confined to a limited number of specially licensed physicians. As a result, the price of heroin smuggled in from Southeast Asia tripled. By 1979, poor weather for crops and increased antidrug enforcement activity choked off the flow of heroin from this region. About the same time, the revolution in Iran that led to the toppling of the monarchy and the beginning of much disorder in that country permitted Iranian heroin to fill the drug void. The subsequent increased supply, decreased price, and decline in social taboos against heroin use fostered a growing black market in imported heroin in the United Kingdom.

Today, heroin abuse in Great Britian is found mostly among the country's unemployed and young people. According to the London *Times*, the Wirral area of Merseyside, Liverpool, a seaport town on the western coast of England, suffers the worst addiction rate in the United Kingdom. There, heroin is the most popular drug among unemployed, poor, and wealthy drug abusers. Out of a population of 338,000, the newspaper reported, there were 1,600 drug addicts in

1986, 1,300 of whom were heroin addicts. And of the 600 new drug users added to the list each year, 400 are heroin abusers. About 75% of the drug users are aged 16 to 24, and about 80% are unemployed.

In France, where the incidence of AIDS infection among heroin addicts is estimated to be 30%, the government permits free exchanges of used needles for sterilized needles in pharmacies. Yet in the Netherlands, where clean needles have already been available since 1985 (originally as a means of stopping hepatitis B infections among addicts), the rate of infection is also about 30%, according to a Dutch drug-enforcement official quoted in the *New York Times*.

The AIDS epidemic has also struck the addict population in Italy, where more than half of the 100,000 addicts are believed by authorities to be infected with the AIDS virus. Naples, afflicted with the double burden of poverty and an organized crime ring that traffics drugs, has one of the worst drug problems in Italy. Officially, there are 9,000 addicts in

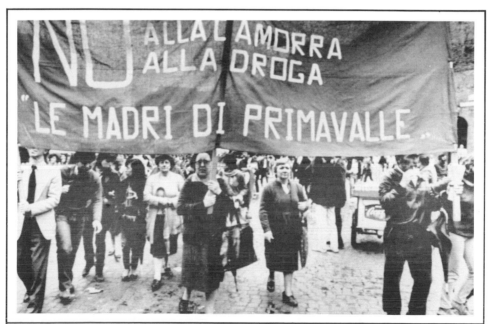

The *"Mothers of Courage"* took to the streets of Rome in 1984 to demonstrate against the Mafia and the illegal drug trade.

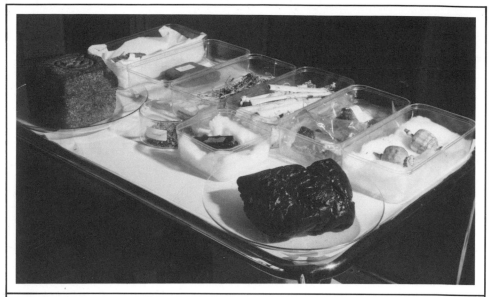

Opium samples taken from different regions by the UN Laboratory in Geneva. The use of heroin has become widespread in Europe, bringing with it a growing crime problem as well as the threat of AIDS.

the city, but some sources say the figure is closer to 20,000. Children not only of the poor but also of wealthy, professional families are becoming addicted to heroin. Tragically, some of the powerful dealers hire children as young as 13 and 14 years old to sell heroin, giving them drugs and paying them as much as $200 or more a week.

In the summer of 1986, a determined band of mothers, furious over the deaths of four youths who died from using adulterated heroin, set out to find and kill the drug dealer who had sold the lethal doses. The dealer escaped, but the women, christened the "Mothers of Courage" by Italian newspapers, formed vigilante groups to chase away drug dealers. They also staged marches to city hall to demand proper drug-rehabilitation facilities, according to the *Dallas Morning News*.

Spanish Loophole Invites Traffickers

Spain has long been a crossroads for Latin American cocaine, Moroccan and Lebanese marijuana and hashish, and Asian heroin entering Europe. In recent years, however, many of these drugs have found a market within Spain — especially since 1983. At that time, Spain decriminalized possession of drugs for personal use, though it did not specify how much would be considered acceptable for personal use.

Drug dealers, faced with a saturated U.S. market, took full advantage of that loophole. According to the Chicago *Tribune*, drug use has soared in Spain, and that country now has the third most serious drug problem in Western Europe, after the Netherlands and Italy.

Among its population of less than 40 million, Spain now has more than 100,000 heroin addicts, according to Spanish police. There are an estimated 30,000 heroin addicts in the Madrid area alone. In fact, some young addicts in Madrid sell hashish on the streets in order to obtain money to buy heroin.

Heroin in Eastern Bloc Countries

In the Soviet Union, the recent surge in narcotic abuse began after the government initiated its anti-alcohol campaign in 1985. Today, glue, hashish, and a crudely processed form of opium called *Koknar*, a sort of heroin substitute, are widely abused.

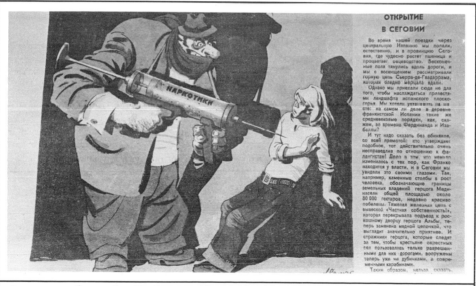

A cartoon from the Soviet weekly Krokodil *satirizes the country's growing narcotics abuse problem.*

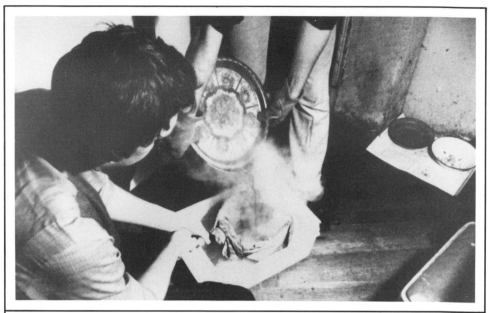

Polish heroin addicts brew kompot, *a liquid containing the boiled-down stems and seedpods of opium plants. The prepared liquid is injected directly into the user's veins for a quick high.*

The source of Koknar is the country's Central Asian region, where both marijuana and opium poppies are grown in abundance. Users boil down the stems and seed pods of poppies and inject the product directly into their veins. The country's militarized border and its network of controls over laboratory equipment and chemicals make large-scale processing of opium into pure heroin virtually impossible. Nevertheless, Koknar abuse has troubled authorities, because the practice led to both addiction and widespread, needle-borne hepatitis in Poland and Hungary during the early 1970s.

In 1987, Interior Minister Aleksandr V. Vlasov declared that official silence on the issue may have contributed to the problem. Since then, the Soviet press has published grim stories of the country's growing narcotic addiction problem. According to Mr. Vlasov, 80% of the users are younger than 30 years old.

The Soviet Union also faces a drug abuse problem among its soldiers fighting the rebels in Afghanistan for control of that country. Soviet soldiers had routinely smoked hashish obtained within Afghanistan, but by the mid-1980s they were also actively abusing heroin sold to them by dealers who were often friendly with the rebels. In this way the rebels used the drug as a source of revenue, while at the same time demoralizing and weakening the Soviet troops.

Elsewhere in the Eastern Bloc, Poland, with a population of about 38 million, has between 200,000 and 600,000 hard drug users and addicts. "The numbers are staggering," Warsaw sociologist Antoni Bielewicz told *Time* magazine in 1987, "and there is no end in sight." In the decaying industrial town of Lodz alone, there are 300 to 400 heroin addicts among a population of 850,000, according to a 1987 report in the *New York Times*. Most of Poland's addicts are under 25 and are hooked on *kompot*, which, like Koknar, is made from poppy stalks and household chemicals. Both the government and the Catholic church there are urging citizens not to abuse drugs and not to sell poppy straw to dealers.

Stimulants, Depressants, and Other Drugs

Stimulants and depressants are widely abused in Europe. In France, where a poll showed that 37% of that country's approximately 54 million people said they suffered from constant anxiety and 57% said they were frequently anxious, sales of anti-anxiety drugs have escalated in the past 15 years. In 1984, these drugs were being prescribed to 49 of every 100 people, compared to 31 in Germany, 23 in Britain, and 13 in the United States.

The *New York Times* reported in 1986 that 8 million French men and women use tranquilizing drugs (not including antidepressants and sleeping pills). The newspaper pointed out that, with psychiatry and psychoanalysis still somewhat taboo in France, people tend to combat their neuroses and sorrows by consuming alcohol and tranquilizers.

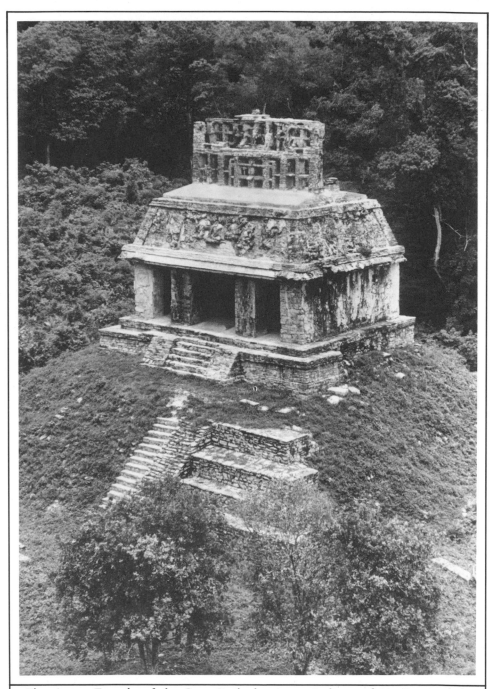

The Aztec Temple of the Sun. Both the Aztec Indians of Mexico and the Incas of Peru permitted alcohol consumption during religious rituals and social celebrations, but discouraged its use at other times.

CHAPTER 5

USE AND ABUSE IN THE AMERICAS

Long before Spanish invaders arrived in America, the Aztec Indians of Mexico and the Incas of Peru had developed and used beverages produced by fermentation. For example, the Aztecs, who had conquered central Mexico by the 15th century, drank *pulque*, a drink fermented from the sap of the maguey, a member of the Amaryllis family (which also includes the aloe, the agave, and the century plant). According to Aztec custom, both drinking and drunkenness among adults was socially sanctioned as an integral part of religious celebrations, agricultural ceremonies, and celebrations of important events in the lives of local leaders. Drinking for the mere sake of drunkenness, however, was discouraged by both the nobility and religious figures.

Soon, however, maguey cultivation expanded to serve a growing population. Taxes on alcoholic beverages became significant sources of revenue and licenses to sell the beverage became more numerous and were sought after for the high profits they secured. Whatever control the ancient Indian nobility had over pulque consumption among the masses decayed as Europeans took control of society. Moreover, the Catholic calendar introduced additional feast days that the Indians celebrated with drink. To a large extent, however, their drunkenness was a response to the shock of the Spanish conquest. Alcohol was an escape from the despair and confusion that followed the destruction of Aztec society.

The History of Alcohol in Latin America

Native fermented beer is also a traditional drink throughout much of Latin America. Despite significant differences in the ingredients and methods of preparation in various areas, the drink is known throughout the region as *chica* ("maize beer"). Chica was a staple commodity during the Inca Empire, which dominated most of the Andean highlands from Colombia southward through Peru and into Chile.

Like the Mexican pulque, chica is enjoyed by Indians of both sexes and all ages. Both beverages also appear to have had symbolic importance in both the religious and political rites of the Mayas of Mesoamerica — the southern part of what is now Mexico, including the Yucatán peninsula. In addition, the Mayas fermented the bark of a particular tree to produce a distinctive regional beer called *balche*.

European authorities in Peru deprived the Incan nobility of their monopoly on chica taverns during the 16th century, undercutting one of their principal power bases. Rather than stopping alcohol consumption or giving the Europeans tighter control over and more tax money from the natives, however, the seizure of the taverns only led to widespread "moonshining" and a loss of tax revenues.

Production of wine began after the Spanish invaders imported grape vines, presumably to lessen the need to take up valuable cargo space with wine in ships bound for these newly claimed lands. After 1551, wine production was underway in Peru, Bolivia, and Argentina. Brazil and Chile eventually began their own wine industries, but other Latin American countries never developed significant wine production facilities. Also in the 16th century, Hernán Cortés, the Spanish conqueror of Mexico, established the first sugar mill for the production of *aguardiente*, or "cane alcohol."

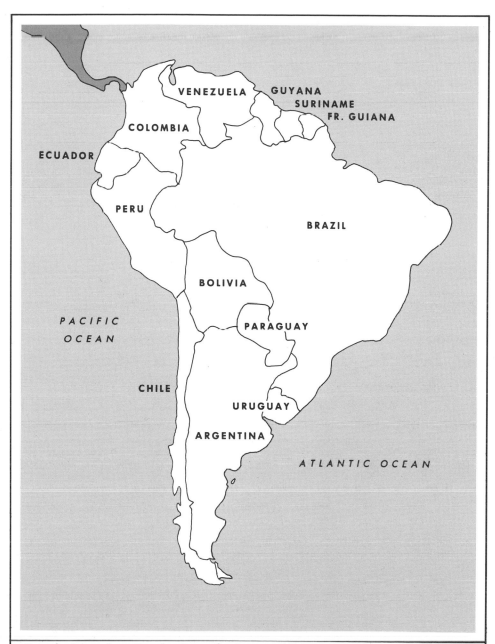

South America. *Production of wine on this continent began in the 16th century and was soon under way in Peru, Bolivia, and Argentina. Brazil and Chile eventually developed wine industries as well.*

How History Affects the Present Day

Despite differences in drinking customs and beverages, one custom of drinking that has remained widespread in Latin American countries is the drinking bout, or group binge. According to a study cited in *Legislative Approaches to Prevention of Alcohol-Related Problems: An Inter-American Workshop*, a characteristic of this custom is that men drink "to the point of stupefaction." Group drinking is an important ritual in itself, without religious significance; solitary drinking is discouraged. This custom has been documented by various researchers in communities throughout the region. Consumption of intoxicating beverages as a way of promoting social cohesion and interrelationship occurs in the Andean countries as well as Central America, Mexico, the lowland

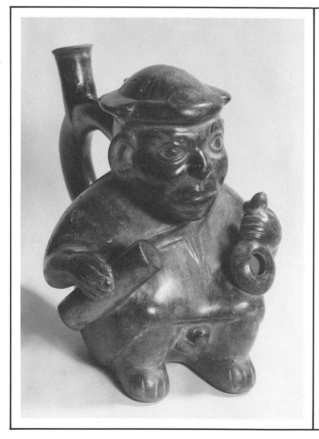

A container used to hold chica, or maize beer. Chica is rich in certain vitamins and calcium and serves as an important nutritional supplement for many poor Latin Americans.

areas of South America, and the Caribbean. Drinking is an important component of fiestas, which are welcome, festive holidays. And in many ethnic cultures, drinking is a ritual that emphasizes equality and solidarity.

In addition, alcoholic beverages are of great economic value as commodities that are both sold and taxed. Researchers have even found alcoholic beverages used as mediums of exchange for paying wages, fines, or taxes in some communities.

Native fermented drinks also play a role in the nutrition of many Latin Americans. A report in the *American Journal of Public Health*, for example, stated that pulque is second only to tortillas as a source of essential vitamins and minerals in the diet of some native communities in central Mexico. Chica, too, is nutritious; it is rich in B-complex and C vitamins as well as calcium, and thus serves as an important food supplement to the typical Andean diet.

In the past, however, use of native fermented drinks, nutritional or not, turned to abuse after the Spanish conquest of the proud Indian cultures. The shock of conquest caused many Indians to seek relief from their distress at being subjugated by abusing a drink traditionally associated with divinity, succor, and social cohesion. Many Indians simply gave up their heritage and drifted into urban areas, where intermarriage with the Spanish produced a burgeoning mestizo (Spanish-Indian) population. Some members of this group grew up with lax or confused patterns of socialization, and without roots in either Indian or Spanish societies.

How the Mestizos Live Today

Mestizos now live in both urban and rural areas. A common element among male mestizos is the desire to achieve the wealth and success of middle- and upper-class Mexicans. But their own lack of skills generally prohibits such upward mobility.

Trapped between their rejection of the simple Indian way of life and their own rejection by the urban upper class they envy, many mestizos find comfort in drinking bouts, during which groups of men consume not only the traditional pulque, but also beer and grain alcohol beverages, especially tequila. As described by researchers in *Beliefs, Behaviors,*

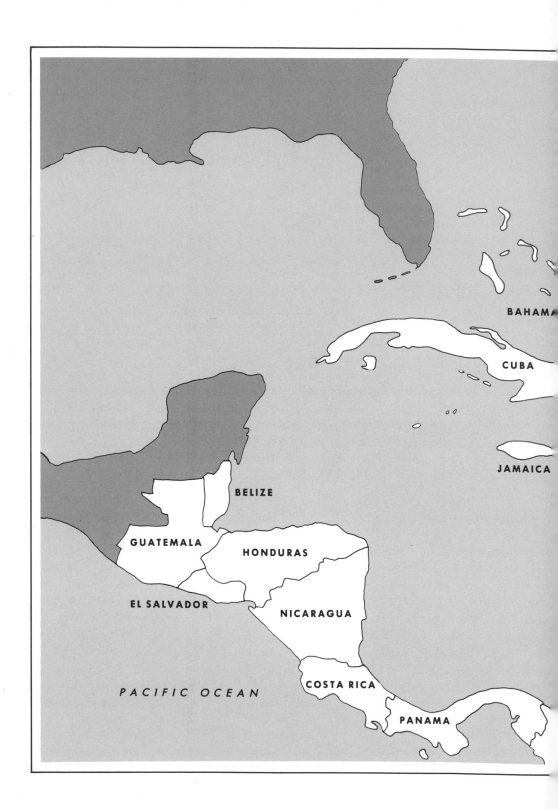

BAHAMA

CUBA

JAMAICA

BELIZE

GUATEMALA

HONDURAS

EL SALVADOR

NICARAGUA

PACIFIC OCEAN

COSTA RICA

PANAMA

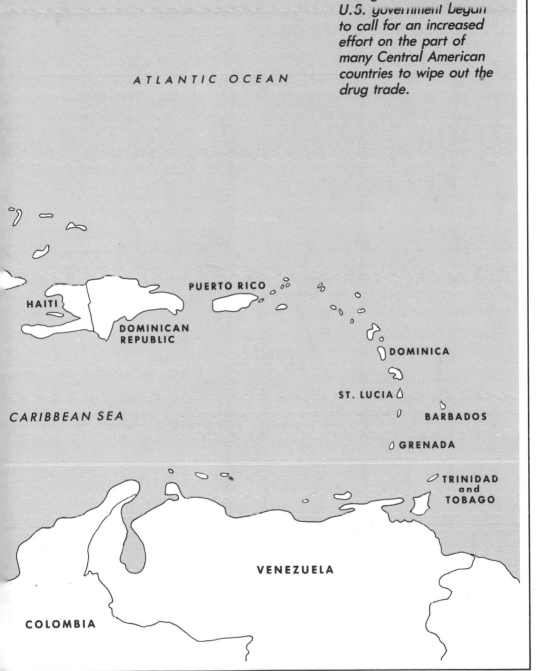

Central America.
During the late 1980s the U.S. government began to call for an increased effort on the part of many Central American countries to wipe out the drug trade.

ATLANTIC OCEAN

PUERTO RICO

HAITI

DOMINICAN REPUBLIC

DOMINICA

ST. LUCIA

CARIBBEAN SEA

BARBADOS

GRENADA

TRINIDAD and TOBAGO

VENEZUELA

COLOMBIA

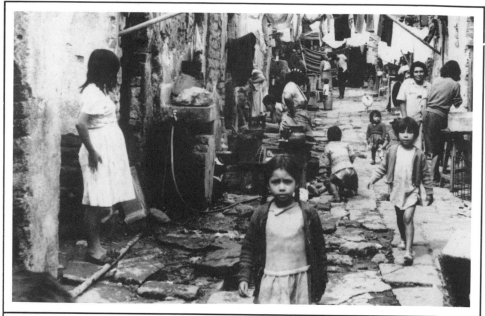

Many mestizos, or people of mixed Spanish-Indian descent, have little sense of cultural identity and are forced by their poverty to live in urban slums, where they often turn to alcohol to escape their despair.

and Alcoholic Beverages: A Cross-Cultural Survey, the mestizo man considers drinking "an essential means of displaying his manly superiority." Both abstinence from alcohol and chronic drunkenness are viewed as signs of weakness. Strength comes from bettering a drinking companion. The need to assert one's *machismo*, or manhood, often leads to insults and fighting, and sometimes to death.

Alcohol and the Upper Classes

Among the middle and upper classes of Mexico, correct drinking behavior is regarded as a social skill; excessive drinking is considered wasteful and destructive. Women generally participate in drinking parties, but for men, drinking still retains a hint of machismo. In this case, however, it reflects the premise that "machismo should be proved not by brute force but by displaying intellectual superiority and sexual prowess," according to Dwight B. Heath of the Inter-American

Workshop. The Mexican upper class as a whole drinks less, and less often, than the rural population.

In contrast to Mexico, members of the upper-middle class in various regions throughout Brazil drink more than do those in the lower class. Drinking among the upper-class Brazilians serves both to symbolize friendship and to demonstrate a cosmopolitan, rather than backward, rural demeanor.

In Argentina, Uruguay, and the southern part of Brazil, recent European immigrants, who brought with them a tradition of sobriety, constitute a sizable majority. Drunkenness in these regions is thus less prevalent than in other parts of South America. As part of their culture, these immigrants — mostly from Spain, Portugal, and Italy — have brought with them both the skills to manufacture, and a preference for, wines rather than the stronger beverages consumed elsewhere on the continent.

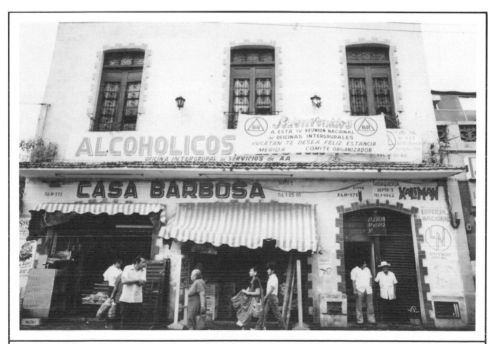

Alcoholics Anonymous (AA) headquarters in Mexico City, Mexico. AA estimates that it has close to 2 million members worldwide, with active groups in 115 different countries.

Alcoholic products available on the international market have become prized in Latin America; treating guests to imported whiskey is often considered a status symbol. Venezuela is the world's largest per-capita importer of alcoholic beverages. Government efforts to curb consumption — for example, through a 15% tax on imported liquor — have been largely unsuccessful.

Home brewing of alcoholic beverages is also widespread throughout Latin America. The unrecorded consumption of home-brewed pulque in Mexico and chica in the Andean countries is paralleled by the manufacture and use of homemade wines in Argentina and Chile. In addition, illegally distilled rum in Chile has long been recognized as contributing to the drinking problem in that country.

Alcohol Abuse in Central and South America

Chile as a whole has a high rate of liver cirrhosis, because of widespread heavy drinking and one of the highest — if not *the* highest—rates of alcoholism in the world.

The consumption of alcoholic beverages starts at a very young age in Chile. According to a study published in 1979 in the *Journal of Studies on Alcohol*, 80% of the 9-year-old children in 2 public and 2 private schools in Santiago occasionally consumed alcohol (usually in the form of a low-alcohol-content sweet beverage), 9% drank daily and 23% drank twice a week.

Alcohol abuse is also a major problem in Brazil. A large proportion of general hospital patients are heavy drinkers, and alcoholism is one of the most frequent diagnoses in Brazilian hospitals.

In Costa Rica, the illegal production of rum made from sugarcane is estimated to equal that of the state liquor monopoly. And studies suggest that in urban Guatemala, heavy, frequent drinking is common among males and females.

Widespread illegal production of alcoholic beverages and the easy availability of legal alcohol have combined with a general acceptance of drinking to establish a formidable challenge to public campaigns aimed at reducing alcohol consumption. Alcohol abuse thus continues to constitute a major public health problem in the region.

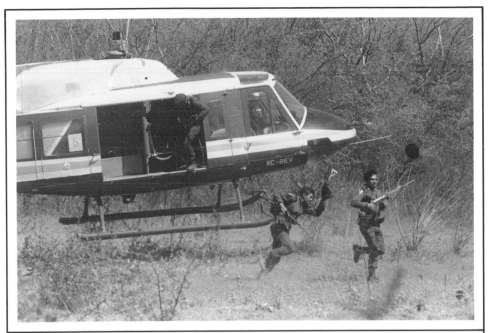

Mexican troops leap from a helicopter during a raid of poppy and marijuana fields in the state of Sinaloa. Despite such efforts Mexico is a major supplier of both marijuana and heroin to the United States.

Mexico: A Major Supplier and User of Marijuana

Mexico, the largest supplier of marijuana to the United States, also has a long tradition of consumption of the drug, both recreationally and as part of religious traditions. For example, members of an Indian tribal group living in communities near the Gulf of Mexico chew the leaves of locally grown marijuana plants as part of their spiritual rituals. According to a folk saying, the herb, called *la santa rosa* (the sacred rose) represents that which is living, "as if it were a small piece of the heart of God." Both male and female priests, as well as their guests, consume *la santa rosa* during ceremonies that are accompanied by music that heightens the visual and auditory hallucinations provoked by the drug.

In addition to the use of marijuana drug within the confines of cultural traditions, outright abuse of the drug is also prevalent. The San Diego *Union* reported in 1987 that Culiacán, the capital of the Mexican state of Sinaloa — a leading producer of marijuana—now has a drug abuse problem.

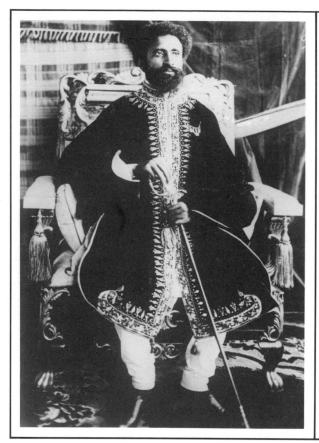

Emperor Haile Selassie of Ethiopia, whose original name was Ras Tafari. Followers of Ras Tafari (Rastafarians) have ritualized the use of marijuana, which they call ganja.

The farmers of this region see the valuable crop as a way out of their poverty. Relatively well-off high school and university students are initially lured into drug use by pushers who give them free "starter samples," according to Dr. Hector Marroquin, the deputy director of public health for the state of Sinaloa.

Sinaloa's problem confirms warnings from many drug experts that any area in the world where drugs are produced illegally for export will eventually find large numbers of its own citizens becoming drug abusers.

Marijuana Use and Abuse in Other Countries

Marijuana has gained in popularity throughout the Americas in large part because of the rising cost of alcohol relative to the price of marijuana. According to the book *Cannabis and*

Culture, edited by Vera Rubin, this has occurred despite deeply rooted cultural differences among the various countries of Latin and South America.

The hemp plant, from which marijuana is derived, is grown in Colombia for both local consumption and export to other countries. In recent years, however, authorities have stepped up their efforts to destroy marijuana fields, as part of an international cooperative effort among drug enforcement agencies to stem the production and export of drugs.

Paraguay is another major producing and trafficking country, shipping out 1,500 to 3,000 metric tons of marijuana annually to countries in South America, especially Brazil and Argentina. More than two tons of Paraguayan marijuana entered Argentina in 1986, for both domestic consumption and export, according to the U.S. State Department's 1987 International Narcotics Control Strategy Report.

Marijuana is also widely consumed in Brazil, although that country apparently does not have a serious problem with abuse of the drug. Among the Tenetchara Indians of the country, the medicine men, called shamans, smoke cannabis to the accompaniment of rhythmic song and dance in a curing ritual that calls upon spirits to aid in healing the sick.

Marijuana as a National Institution

The Caribbean island of Jamaica produces marijuana destined for the United States, despite eradication efforts supported by the U.S. government. But whereas many young Americans think of marijuana smoking as a recreational pastime, to many Jamaicans it is something entirely different: a national institution. According to *Cannabis and Culture*, Jamaicans occasionally smoke marijuana — called *ganja* in their culture — in the form of cigarettes called spliffs. But the most common form of consumption is marijuana tea, which is reputed to have therapeutic properties.

The social importance of cannabis in Jamaica has its roots in the Indian subcontinent. During the late 19th century, East Indian indentured laborers, recruited to replace the emancipated slaves in the sugarcane fields, brought with them the custom of ganja use. Ironically, the great majority of ganja users today are not East Indians — a minority in Jamaica — but rather the rural and urban black laborers descended from the emancipated slaves.

Jamaicans cultivate their own cannabis plants on plots that usually range from 20 to 200 plants, although much larger plots do exist. Growing ganja is an agricultural sideline that supplements the laborers' incomes and ensures a ready supply of the herb.

Major ganja vendors in a community operate "herb camps," which provide a recreational atmosphere complete with alcoholic beverages, music, and sometimes games and television. Less important vendors run "herb yards," which simply provide clients with a place to consume their own ganja or ganja bought from the vendor.

Ganja consumption is a lifelong custom that begins when parents give their infants and young children ganja tea, which is thought to be helpful in preventing disease. Adolescent boys smoke ganja sporadically, usually obtaining it from young vendors rather than from adults. The practice is considered a rite of passage into adulthood.

Adults tend to smoke more often. Ganja is more accessible to them, both because they have a steady income with which to buy it and because many adults cultivate small plots

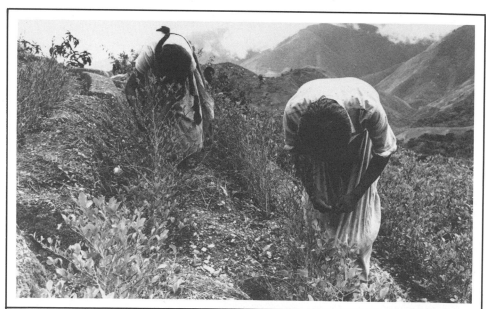

Bolivian women cultivate coca shrubs. Since ancient times the Indians of Bolivia and Peru have chewed coca leaves to give them energy.

for their own use. Older people smoke less for a variety of reasons. Their incomes are low, they are less physically able to cultivate their own ganja plots, and, with age, they have often lost their smoking companions to death.

Many laborers use ganja to increase their work capacity. According to *Cannabis and Culture*, "Ganja, in the rural reaches of Jamaica, is a substance that apparently permits the individual to face, start, and carry through the most difficult and distasteful manual labor." Although the upper classes look down on ganja consumption, among the laborers smoking symbolizes camaraderie, equality, and belonging.

Jamaican adherents of the Rastafarian faith have ritualized the use of ganja. Followers of Ras Tafari, who later changed his named to Haile Selassie when he was crowned emperor of Ethiopia, Rastafarians are generally a peaceful people. Some members of the religion, however, have become involved in the often violent marijuana trade in Miami, New York, New Jersey, and in Hartford, Connecticut.

Cocaine: The Ancient Drug of Choice

The coasts, highlands, and rain forests of South America abound in species of plants known to alter normal, waking consciousness. Use of the coca plant, *Erythroxylon coca*, from which cocaine is derived, has been dated from as early as 2500 B.C.E.

Indians in the Andes Mountains of Bolivia and Peru have long chewed the leaves of the coca plant for their stimulant effects. The drug helps them cope with life in the high altitudes, where hard work and hunger are staples of everyday existence. And in some tribes, coca leaves have been used in conjunction with hallucinogenic plants as part of ritual healing ceremonies.

By 1980, many Americans had tired of marijuana and adopted cocaine as their drug of choice. The long cultural history of coca use in South America took a destructive and bloody turn when drug traffickers discovered the huge American market for cocaine waiting to be exploited.

The wealth and violence of Colombian traffickers, who have killed scores of judges, journalists, and police who defied them, have triumphed over the cooperative efforts of U.S. and Colombian drug officials to stem the flow of cocaine from

Colombia into the United States. And as severe as the problems of violence, crime, and corruption that arise from drug trafficking are in Colombia, they are only a part of the drug menace threatening that country.

In the past, cocaine traffickers obtained their coca paste from Peru and Bolivia and processed it into cocaine for distribution abroad. But during the late 1970s, Colombian drug dealers tried to grow their own coca plants in the mountains of northern and western Colombia. These crops were inferior to the imported strain and not suitable for processing into the white powder sold in the United States and Europe. To add to this problem, wholesale prices began to drop during the 1980s.

Faced with this threat to their profits, the Colombian dealers turned their own people into addicts by supplying them with this inferior brand of cocaine. The dealers mixed their surplus dark oily coca paste with tobacco to produce *bazuco*, a cigarette that gives a quick, intense high, followed by a craving for more of the drug.

Bazuco traffickers targeted Colombia's marijuana smokers, almost giving the drug away at first to get consumers addicted. The paste contains high amounts of the active ingredient, but it also contains dangerously large quantities of kerosene, gasoline, ether, and other chemicals used in the coca-paste refining process. Thus, in addition to its high addiction potential, bazuco also poses a serious toxic hazard to its users.

Unfortunately, this hazard has not curbed the rate of addiction. Bazuco use has now spread from low-income groups into the middle class. By 1986, according to the Dallas *Times Herald*, 600,000 young Colombians were hooked on bazuco, which experts in that country said was "frying the brains" of a whole generation.

The coca paste problem is now threatening Peru, where the concoction is called *keke*. Coca cultivation increased during late 1985 and early 1986, according to the United Nations' 1986 report of the International Narcotics Control Board. The tendency to move cocaine-processing facilities closer to the areas of cultivation has increased the amount of paste and cocaine available for consumption by the local population.

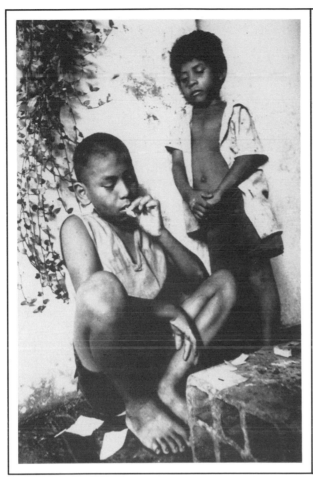

A Peruvian boy smokes a bazuco, a cigarette containing coca paste. Bazuco contains dangerously large quantities of the kerosene, gasoline, and ether used in the coca-refining process and poses a serious toxic hazard to its users.

As in other parts of South America, hunger, poverty, and a surplus of contaminated coca paste have nurtured a growing number of coca-paste cigarette addicts in Bolivia, where the product is known as *pitillo*. There drug traffickers hire peasants to stomp the coca leaves into paste. As part of their pay, the workers, both children and adults, receive free pitillo. This strategy ensures an endless supply of addicted laborers eager to work for both money and drugs.

According to the *Dallas Morning News*, government officials in La Paz estimated in 1986 that there were about 100,000 addicts in Bolivia, out of a population of 5.6 million. The number was growing, they said, "at alarming rates." And as in other countries where drug abuse is severe, there are charges that police corruption contributes to the problem.

Ecuador also faces a cocaine abuse problem. Like Peru and Bolivia, Ecuador has been mainly a transit country for coca derivatives. But in recent years, extensive areas have come under coca cultivation. Despite destruction of many fields and dismantling of laboratories, the country now faces "soaring increases" in the abuse of coca paste, according to the 1986 report of the International Narcotics Control Board.

Brazil's cocaine abuse problem is not serious compared to that of Colombia, Peru, and Bolivia. But family and personal problems drive some middle-class youths to drugs, especially hashish. Among the underclasses, which cannot afford drugs, youths are driven by hunger, poverty, and squalor to sniff gasoline, for example, or use medications that have been diverted from legal use.

In addition, the country's strategic importance to cocaine traffickers has turned Brazil into a major processing and transshipment point. The country is the only South American nation that sells, in industrial quantities, the ether and acetone needed to turn coca base into cocaine. Now that Brazilian authorities have made it difficult to ship the chemicals out of the country, traffickers ship coca paste and coca base through Bolivia to Brazil for processing there in clandestine laboratories. Brazilian authorities, concerned that the cocaine trade will spill over into its own communities, have already established drug-abuse prevention campaigns around the country.

The problem could become acute in the 430 slums of São Paulo, which are home to 1.5 million people. Many of the slums near the city's affluent, cocaine-consuming section are controlled by drug bosses. These criminals have become heroes to many of the people by providing jobs for youths who sell marijuana and cocaine, chasing away outside criminals, and discouraging police from entering the slums.

A similar scenario is being played out in the Bahamas, which serves as a way station for marijuana and cocaine shipped from South America to the United States. Government corruption and misguided support of traffickers by the local population has led, as in Colombia and Brazil, to a burgeoning cocaine abuse epidemic. Although the two major political parties in the Bahamas disagree on many other issues, both have stated that drug abuse is the most serious problem facing that country today. Indeed, the flood of drugs and escalating addiction rate prompted the leader of an antidrug group called the National Drug Council to tell the *Wall Street Journal*, "Cocaine is wiping out our young people."

By 1987, Nassau alone had about 100 "base houses" serving up *cokomoe*, the Bahamian name for crack, to both youths and adults. According to a report in Florida's *Orlando Sentinel*, in that year alone there were about 6,000 Bahamian crack addicts out of a population of 225,000.

The newspaper also reported that most of the patients at Sandilands Rehabilitation Hospital in Nassau have been unaware how much more addictive crack is than regular cocaine. Most patients in the hospital are between 18 and 30 years old, but addicts as young as 9 and as old as 60 have been treated there. Space is limited, however, and even the hospital's chief nurse admitted to the newspaper that the recovery rate is minimal. "The Bahamas is small," she said. "They go back to their neighborhoods and their friends are there waiting to give them the stuff for free. The temptation is great."

Hallucinogens and Spirituality

Before their conquest by Spanish invaders the Aztec Indians of Mexico worshipped three plants that contained hallucinogenic substances: *Teonancatl*, a mushroom; *ololiuqui*, a vine belonging to the morning-glory family; and a cactus called *peyote*.

Peyote, whose active ingredient is mescaline, was the most important of these plants; the Indians called it the "flesh of the gods." Spanish priests, however, called peyote the devil's root, banned its use, and drove the practice of using it underground.

The cult of the sacred mushroom exists today in the southern Mexican state of Oaxaca, where healers partake of the mushroom alone or in the company of the person they are helping. The various species of hallucinogenic Mexican mushrooms, *Psilocybe mexicana*, *P. zapotecorum*, and *P. caeruluscens*, all contain psilocybin and psilocin, which induce visions and trances that the cultists believe empower the healer to diagnose and cure diseases, according to *Hallucinogens: Cross-Cultural Perspectives*.

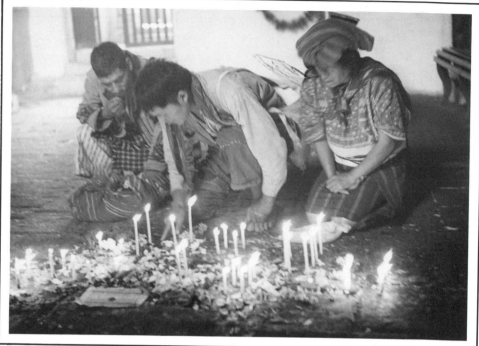

A Guatemalan peyote ceremony. Peyote was called "flesh of the gods" by the Aztecs and is still used in religious ceremonies by indigenous peoples in both North and South America.

Indians and urban mestizo populations in the tropical rain forests of Peru, Colombia, and Brazil use the woody *ayahuasca* vines as an integral part of folk healing. The ayahuasca vines, which include various species of *Banisteriopsis*, contain alkaloids (especially harmine, harmaline, and tetrahydroharmaline) that make these plants powerful hallucinogens. In the Peruvian Amazon region, especially, folk healers called *ayahuasqueros* consume a drink prepared from the vine during the ritual curing of those illnesses that are mostly emotional or psychological in origin.

The ritual also occurs in urban areas, including the Amazon city of Iquitos, where the folk healing practices represent a complex mix of modern medicine, tribal Indian beliefs, and a bit of Roman Catholic theology. The drug does not serve as a panacea for illness, but rather as one part of a complex healing ceremony.

On the Peruvian north coast, specialized healers called *maestros* use hallucinogenic plants to cure patients of diseases thought to be caused by witchcraft. The most commonly used plant is the San Pedro cactus (*Trichocereus pachanoi*), which contains mescaline. Cut up and boiled with various additives, the cactus is used as an agent whose effect will reveal to the maestro the source of the bewitchment.

Shamans among the Desána tribe in northwest Colombia routinely induce ecstatic trances in themselves with powerful plant hallucinogens, especially *yagé*, which is identical to the ayahuasca of the Peruvian Andes.

South American Indians also discovered the psychoactive properties of many other species of plants, which are used alone or as additives to heighten or otherwise modify the metaphysical experience of the shaman. Among them are particularly potent snuffs derived from seeds of the plants *Anadenanthera peregrina* and *A. colubrina* and from the inner bark of trees of the genus *Virola*.

The Yanomama Indians of the upper Orinoco River in Venezuela use intoxicating snuff made from Virola bark; the effects of the snuff, however, are activated by adding certain other plant materials to the concoction. Their sophisticated knowledge of the pharmacology of native plant life suggests that South American Indians have been experimenting with psychoactive plant drugs for many years. In support of this theory, archaeological evidence shows that the ritual use of the mescaline-containing San Pedro cactus stretches back more than 3,000 years.

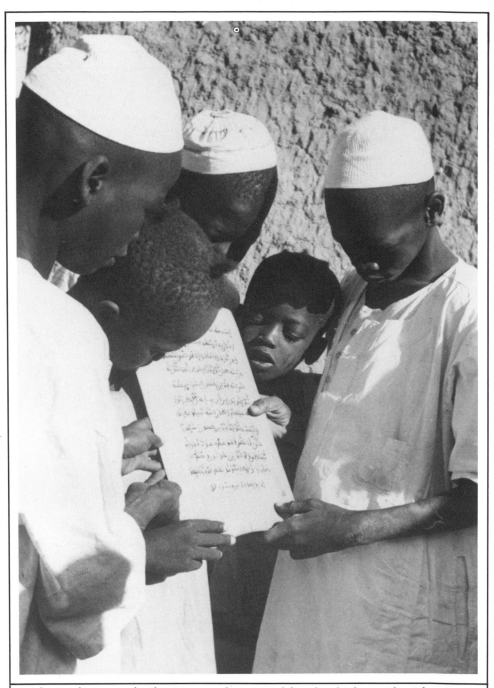

African boys study the Koran, the sacred book of Islam. The Islamic religion, widely practiced in the Middle East and Africa, strictly forbids gambling and drinking alcohol.

CHAPTER 6

USE AND ABUSE IN THE MIDDLE EAST AND AFRICA

The Islamic religion, widely practiced in the Middle East as well as by people in various countries throughout the world, strictly forbids gambling and drinking alcohol. In Iran, for example, after a militantly Islamic regime came to power following a revolution in 1979, the government prohibited drinking. Nevertheless, according to the *International Journal of the Addictions* (1986), some people still manage to obtain liquor or make alcoholic drinks at home.

In Iran, alcohol consumers drink mostly hard liquor, rather than fortified drinks such as sherry. Beer is often drunk before proceeding to hard liquor. Table wine is not a favorite among either Iranian men or women but Iranian Jews produce a high-alcohol homemade wine for their own consumption.

Israel, on the other hand, does not prohibit alcohol, although the Jews have traditionally drunk in moderation, if at all. In the 1980s, however, there is a growing concern over alcohol abuse among Israelis. According to Professor David Krasilowsky, director of Israel's Talbia Psychiatric Hospital, the growing problem of alcohol abuse in that country reflects the nation's ongoing conflict with its neighbors, economic

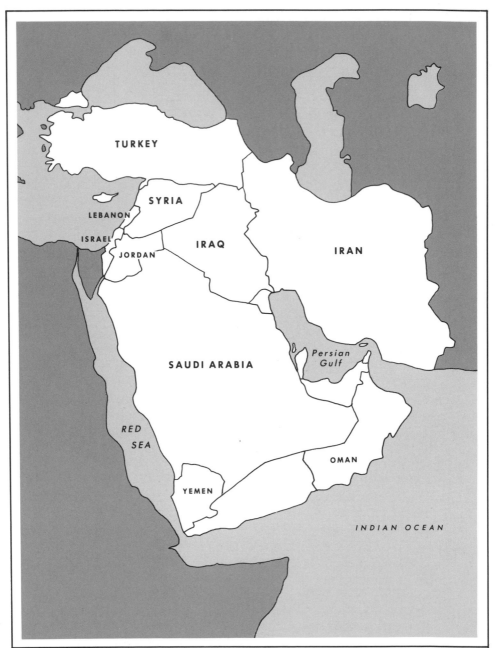

The Middle East. There has been increased concern expressed over the growing alcohol abuse problem in Israel, which many believe may be partly attributable to the nation's ongoing conflicts with its neighbors.

difficulties, and the problems of Jewish refugees from abroad trying to adapt to their new homeland.

During his speech at the 1985 International Congress on Alcohol Dependence held in Jerusalem, Dr. Krasilowsky warned that unless preventive steps are taken, there is good reason to be alarmed over the increasing consumption of alcohol by Israeli youths. During that same conference, Pnina Eldar, director of Israel's Alcoholism Treatment and Prevention Program, reported that 20% of Israeli teenagers drink wine once a week or 3 to 4 times a month; they consume beer almost every day.

Disrupted African Beer Traditions

Alcohol has a long social history in East Africa, where locally brewed beer has enhanced social functions for centuries. Beer drinking has long been important in village life, especially to break the monotony when people are not working, according to *Beliefs, Behaviors, and Alcoholic Beverages*. Beer once cemented business deals, embellished brides' dowries, and was offered to tribal chiefs as a tribute.

Invading Europeans disrupted this traditional pattern of alcohol consumption. Although white invaders had raided Africa for centuries to obtain slaves, it was not until the 19th century that they began to carve out empires for themselves on the continent. The Europeans who settled in Africa brought with them distilled liquor, in the form of rum, gin, and whiskey. Eventually, many Africans turned to these "modern" drinks and away from the traditional beer fermented or distilled from bananas or other native crops. In some tribes, this shift from the traditional fruit beers to the harder spirits disrupted their way of life.

The social disruption of the Bantu tribes of southern Africa was a dramatic case in point. The Bantu, already suffering from some cultural upheaval because of the influx of Europeans, succumbed to the temptations of the new drinks. The invaders produced large amounts of poor quality wine and hard liquor that were unfit for export, and in order to dispose of their products, the Europeans gave black laborers wine as part of their wages. The finer European liquors also found many customers among the native Africans through the underground market.

The breakdown of Bantu society, awash in European alcoholic drinks that were often consumed in the absence of Bantu social constraints, led to the dissolution of Bantu culture and families. In the 19th and early 20th centuries, many Bantu men drifted to urban centers and diamond mines to find employment and liquor. Prostitution and violence flourished, and both women and children patronized local drinking establishments.

Drinking Styles in South Africa

South Africa also has a long history of alcohol use, although there are distinct ethnic differences in drinking styles among its peoples. The traditional drink of native South African blacks is nutritious beer brewed from sorghum. Although initially prohibited, European liquor soon became available and added to the blacks' options. Black South African men still drink mostly beer, and although many prefer malt beer, sorghum beer is still the most popular drink, according to a 1983 report in the *Journal of Studies on Alcohol*. Two-thirds of black women questioned said they abstained from drinking, but the report suggests that the social stigma attached to drinking by women might have persuaded some women who used alcohol to deny it.

The white population of South Africa has consumed wine since settlers first began planting grape vines there in the 17th century. Today, white men consume mostly malt beer, and white women mostly wine. Alcohol use is widely regarded as a good way to relax and as an acceptable social lubricant. Thus, moderate drinking is the norm, and both heavy drinking and total abstinence are considered antisocial.

Among the group known as Coloreds — people of mixed European and native South African descent — men drink mainly wine, according to the journal's report, and colored women drink both wine and malt beer. However, like the black women, nearly two-thirds of the colored women denied drinking any alcohol. Drinking among the colored population is considered to be an important factor responsible for the "economic and physical deterioration of a considerable section" of this group, according to the report. Black and colored drinking occurs mostly on weekends, possibly because so many of the workers in this group are paid on Fridays.

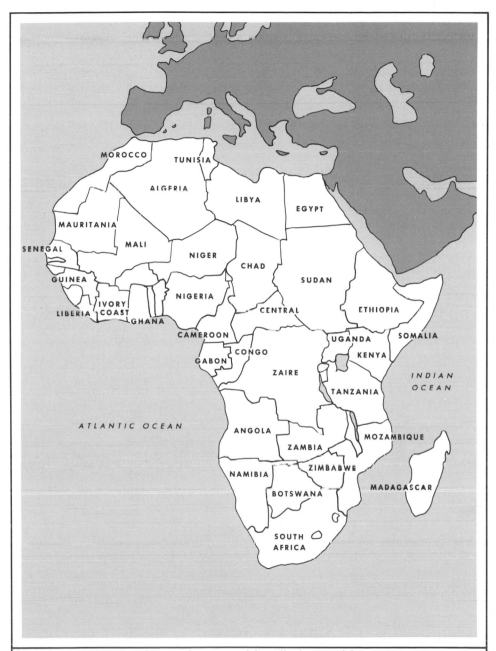

Africa. Although Africans have used locally brewed beer to enhance social gatherings for centuries, European settlers introduced many natives to hard liquor with unsettling results.

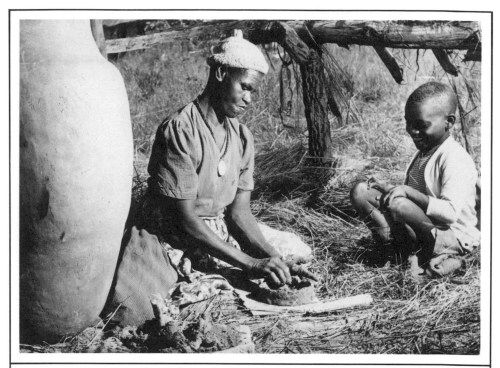

Nauma Mai Guta, an African artisan, displays the technique she uses to create her pottery. Guta formerly brewed beer from bananas or other native crops and sold it to support her children.

East Africa's Drinking Problem

Excessive drinking is widespread throughout East Africa. In Nairobi, Kenya, as many as 46% of male heads of households in a slum area near that city and 24% of female heads of households were alcoholics. Most alcoholics did not participate in community activities, and heavy drinking was associated with cannabis smoking, as well as prostitution, theft, and other forms of antisocial activity. The alcohol problem has been exacerbated by permissive laws that make alcohol readily available to both adults and children. Alcohol is also heavily advertised, which may contribute to the problem.

The Khat Chewers of the Red Sea

Long before Western drugs took hold in the area around the Red Sea, people chewed the small, serrated, bitter leaves and young shoots of an indigenous plant variously called *khat, kat, qaat*, or *gat*. The leaf of this small, whitish tree, *Catha edulis*, contains cathinone, a substance chemically and pharmacologically related to amphetamine.

Khat chewing is an old, traditional habit in this area, which includes such countries as Yemen, Ethiopia, and Djibouti. Its stimulating and euphoric effects prompt users to spend much time foraging for the plant in this hot, harsh corner of the world.

According to an account in the *New York Times Magazine*, when a typical male khat user wakes up in the morning he is lethargic and in low spirits. After breakfast, he contemplates his miseries — uncertain health, the burden of raising a family — before staggering into the field to gather khat. There, with a gourd of water, he sips and chews for two or three hours, until his spirits soar and he feels a surge of energy. Rejuvenated by his khat, he works for several hours until he is exhausted. After an afternoon meal, he remembers his miseries again, and goes back to his khat tree.

Hashish Helps Egyptian Poor Get By

Hashish smoking in Egypt is a centuries-old custom that has survived civil laws and religious prohibition. Although laws against its use stretch back to the 14th century, and one Egyptian official banned its use in 1940, today cannabis remains the most popular intoxicant in Egypt.

The traditional Islamic prohibition of alcohol leads some hashish users to feel superior to alcoholics, as well as to consumers of other drugs such as opium and cocaine. Nevertheless, cannabis use in Egypt is most widespread among the poor working class, who have themselves traditionally been held in contempt by the upper classes.

Today, much of the hashish distributed throughout the large cities of Egypt, most notably Cairo, comes from Lebanon. In Cairo, according to a 1980 *New York Times* report, flourishing wholesale and retail drug markets provide jobs for youths. In the winding alleys and cul de sacs of Cairo's Batanniya market, merchants deal openly in hashish and opium. Lookouts posted in this maze sound alarms well before police can make raids.

Many hashish shipments arriving from abroad are hidden in tombs in cemeteries on the outskirts of Cairo, according to the same report. On occasion, sham funerals take place.

At the point where, according to Muslim tradition, the body is removed from the coffin and placed in the grave, hashish is distributed instead.

Cannabis is also produced and used throughout the African continent, according to the 1986 report of the United Nations' International Narcotics Control Board. Much of the drug is also shipped to Western Europe, primarily from Morocco but increasingly from Ghana and Nigeria.

Cannabis Use Among the Moroccan Rif

Despite Roman and Arab invasions since ancient times, the Berbers of the mountain and pastoral regions of Morocco and Algeria continue to speak their own language. The Berber culture was disrupted, however, during the Spanish colonial period from 1912 to 1956, when vast areas of land were denuded of forests. Although the land was cleared so that it could be cultivated and the trees used for fuel, deforestation rendered the area unsuitable for anything but dry farming of

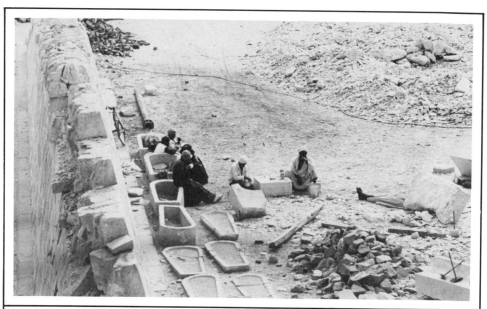

Hashish shipments arriving from abroad are often hidden in tombs in cemeteries on the outskirts of Cairo, Egypt. On these occasions sham funerals take place, and hashish is distributed to those who attend.

grains and fruits — and the cultivation of *Cannabis sativa*, a species of marijuana known locally as *kif*

The Spanish extracted whatever they could from this fragile land while fighting off rebels in the Rif Mountains, which ring the northern part of Morocco. Throughout the years of exploitation and poverty, according to *Cannabis and Culture*, kif remained an important cash crop among the Berbers of the Rif Mountains as well as a stimulant among Rif tribal groups.

Although kif is illegal, the Berbers do not consider it evil, and, unlike alcohol, there is no religious prohibition of its use. The cultivation and distribution networks are well entrenched and serve as important economic lifelines in this poor region. Moreover, legal sanctions are minimal, when enforced at all, and certain cafes cater exclusively to kif smokers, who grind the drug and mix it with tobacco.

Unlike in Western countries, where marijuana smoking is often a sign of youthful rebellion, kif smoking among the Berbers is largely restricted to middle-aged men. Young rebels are more likely to drink beer or wine. The educated elite consider kif smoking a mark of the poor, illiterate, and backward, and also prefer to consume alcohol.

Kif smoking does not seem to be associated with mysticism or with religious rituals. Rather, it a source of pleasure and an escape from the daily depression and anxiety experienced by the natives of this harsh land.

Heroin: The Nigerian Connection

Until recently, heroin was virtually unknown in Africa. Now both the island nation of Mauritius and the West African country of Nigeria serve as transit points for heroin originating in India, Pakistan, Afghanistan, and Thailand and bound for the United States. Like Latin America, with its growing population of cocaine addicts, these heroin-exporting countries now have a growing population of heroin addicts. Other transit countries in Africa, such as the Ivory Coast and Ghana in West Africa, now also risk the same fate.

Nigerian smugglers have become especially active in bringing heroin into Western countries. But not all the heroin coming into Nigeria is consumed or smuggled out. According

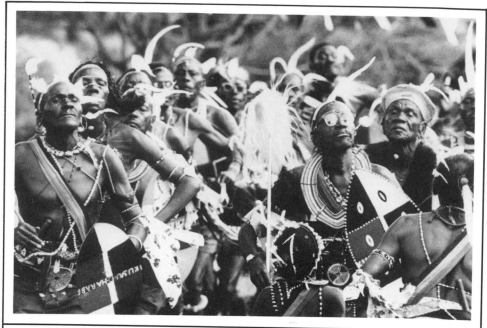

Kenyans perform a tribal dance for American visitors. Modernization has undermined many African traditions, causing a number of social problems, substance abuse among them.

to the U.S. State Department's "International Narcotics Control Strategy Report" for March 1987, some heroin is traded for cocaine flown in directly from Brazil and Colombia. And like the imported heroin, some of the cocaine is abused by Nigerians themselves.

Hallucinogens and the Fang's Cultural Crash

The Fang tribal group of Zaire, in the northwest portion of that equatorial African country, responded to the shock of 19th-century French colonization by adapting a religious movement called the Bwiti cult to its own needs. With their own way of life disrupted, the Fang sought to reestablish social cohesion in their ancient society by combining the rituals and beliefs of nearby Bantu peoples with those of the original Bwiti cult of tribes in neighboring central Gabon. Christian symbols brought in by the Europeans also found their way into this religious amalgam.

By the end of the 19th century, the Fang had added to their Bwiti rituals the use of the plant *Tabernanthe iboga*, which contains the hallucinogenic alkaloids tabernanthine, ibogaine, and iboluteine. Formerly used to relieve fatigue and aid in hunting, the plant now serves as a means to induce visions of the Bwiti divinity, and to attain superior knowledge of life.

As part of the hallucinogenic experience, the initiate is expected to see the Bwiti divinity. According to the description of the Bwiti cult rituals detailed in *Hallucinogens: Cross-Cultural Perspectives*, by Marlene Dobkin De Rios, "the expectation of seeing the Bwiti divinity structures the nature of the given subjective hallucinogenic experience, so that most, if not all, candidates claim to see this power, real or imagined."

If a candidate fails to see the divinity, however, "he is given repeated doses of iboga, a procedure which probably kills both him and his doubts."

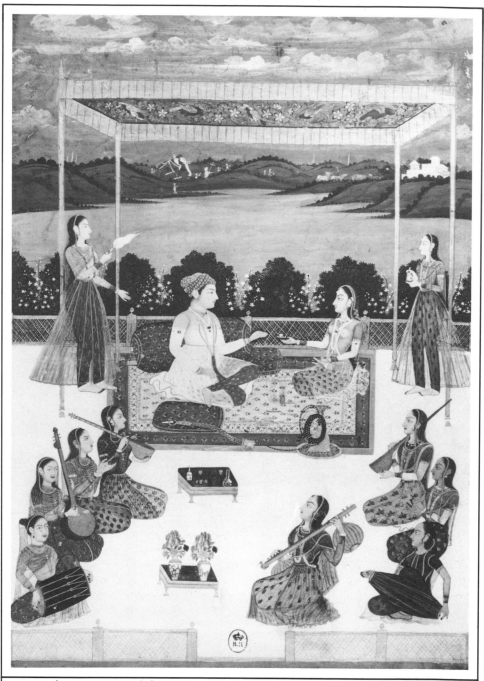

An Indian miniature depicts a man and a woman enjoying an afternoon beverage and some entertainment. Many ancient Indian aristocrats enjoyed somarasa, an alcoholic drink introduced by Aryan invaders.

CHAPTER 7

USE AND ABUSE IN ASIA

About 2000 B.C.E., the Aryans ("noble ones") swooped down from the Himalayas into India, invading an already thriving civilization of dark-skinned people of Australoid origin. The Aryans brought with them their taste for *somarasa*, the juice of a mysterious plant called *soma*, and *sura*, a distilled spirit probably manufactured from rice. Aristocrats and warriors consumed the liquor, as did some common people, who used it in certain religious rituals. But beyond this limited use, consumption of alcohol was frowned upon by Indian society.

When the British colonized India in the 18th century, however, alcohol use slowly spread — to the middle classes, to Indians drafted into the imperial services of Britain, to the power elite, and, to some extent, to industrial workers. Revenue from taxes on liquor further solidified the drug's hold on Indian society. Despite this creeping popularity of alcohol, India was very much a "dry" country, relative to Western cultures. Even before India won its independence from Great Britain, social reformers and political leaders, including Mohandas K. Gandhi, considered alcohol consumption to be a social evil and urged a ban on drinking.

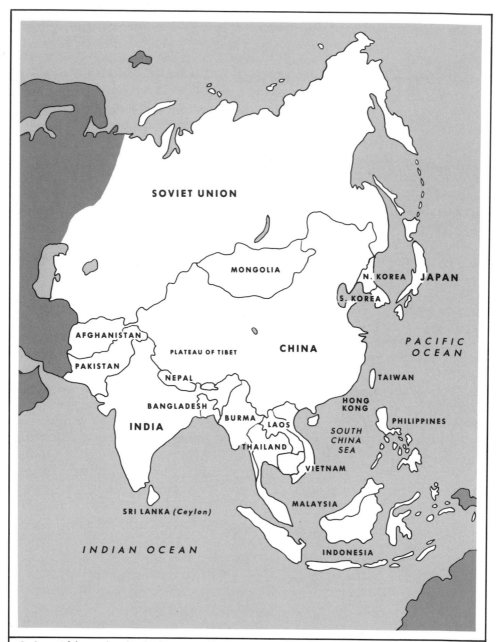

Asia. Although alcohol is usually consumed only in moderation in China and the alcoholism rate there remains low, both India and Japan are now faced with growing alcohol abuse problems.

When India became independent in 1947, Article 47 of its constitution declared the government's intention to enforce the prohibition of alcohol. Today, however, India's state governments violate this edict, in large part because of the tax revenues alcohol generates. According to the *New York Times*, there were more than 200 brands of whiskey, 50 brands of rum, 30 types of brandy, and 50 varieties of beer being produced in India. A top anti-alcohol and drug-enforcement official called liquor "the most widely abused drug in the country."

A spokesman for the liquor industry claimed that nearly half of the national liquor production was "country," or cheap, rumlike liquor made from sugar. Regardless of the source, the dramatic increase in consumption of distilled liquor has had serious economic and social consequences.

Alcohol was formerly fermented at home from spare agricultural products, and thus there was a limited quantity available. Moreover, the alcohol content never reached more than 4 to 5%, and use was occasional and recreational. Now, however, alcohol appears to be replacing cannabis and opium as the favorite drug for festive occasions, according to a 1984 report in *Impact of Science on Society*. Although most prevalent among males, alcohol use is also spreading among educated urban women in middle and upper socioeconomic groups and among students.

Many of India's rural poor spend their precious surplus farm income on alcohol. Heavy consumption of high-alcohol-content beverages has also led to an increase in road accidents, machine and farm equipment accidents, and violent crime. Family life has suffered, and there has been increasing poverty, debt, and mortgaging of property to raise money to buy alcoholic beverages.

The change in drinking habits has also led to a dramatic increase in the incidence of alcoholism, as well as deaths from drinking adulterated homemade beverages. Not all customs have disappeared, however. Drinking is still prohibited to the Brahmans, who are members of the highest caste of the Hindu religion.

The Indian Council of Medical Research reported in 1985 that 20% of city drinkers had become alcoholics and that the rate of alcoholism among drinkers in some villages was as high as 30 to 40%. In response to the rising tide of alcohol abuse, the All India Prohibition Council has worked over the past 50 years to enforce prohibition and encourage abstinence.

In 1980, the T. T. Ranganathan Clinical Research Foundation was established to offer treatment to alcoholics. The center was named after a young man who died of alcoholism at the age of 33. The foundation has helped to dispel the burden of guilt among the families of alcoholics and to educate the Indian public on the nature of alcoholism as a disease, rather than an evil weakness.

Wine Drinking in China: Yesterday and Today

Observations and scientific surveys of the drinking habits of Chinese in the People's Republic of China, Taiwan, New York, and Hong Kong consistently show that this ethnic group has a much lower rate of alcohol abuse and alcoholism than that found in people native to Western countries. No matter where the Chinese live, it seems, if their culture remains intact they tend to avoid raucous drinking bouts and public displays of drunkenness. Not all Chinese share this aversion to alcohol abuse, of course, especially as Western influence is modifying Chinese behavior.

Moreover, ancient Chinese poems betray an enthusiasm for alcohol, which is usually referred to as "wine," regardless of the method of production. The earliest wines, such as rice wine, were made from grains, for grapes were not imported into China until around 200 B.C.E., and beer brewing was not introduced until the mid-19th century.

Today, the People's Republic of China is permitting several European and American companies to set up wine-producing facilities to produce red and white wine as well as brandy, both for internal consumption and export. The current interest in wine is more reminiscent of ancient China than of Chinese attitudes toward the beverage during the past several centuries.

Today, Chinese drinking habits tend more to moderation. The low rate of alcohol abuse and alcoholism is a matter for speculation, but, according to the book *Beliefs, Behaviors, and Alcoholic Beverages*, of special note is the "traditional Chinese socio-cultural structure, informed by Confucian phi-

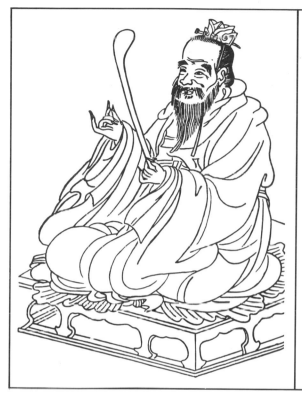

A drawing of the ancient Chinese philosopher Confucius, who is credited with saying "Drinking knows no limit, but never be boisterous with drinking."

losophy, which proscribes excesses, teaches propriety in interpersonal behavior, and stresses intellectual control rather than emotional display."

Confucius was a Chinese philosopher who lived from 551 to 479 B.C.E.. Confucius taught many different ethics and virtues. He believed that if the ruler of a country is good, then his people will imitate and respect him, and those people living in troubled countries will come to his country. In this way, the country will grow and be powerful.

Among the many virtues Confucius taught were loyalty, faithfulness, wisdom, righteousness, and self-cultivation. Confucius also stressed *li*, the rules of proper conduct expected from all gentlemen, *ren*, or benevolent love, and the maxim "Do not do unto others what you would not like yourself." In accordance with his teachings of controlled, polite, and courtly behavior, Confucius is said to have warned that "drinking knows no limit, but never be boisterous with drinking."

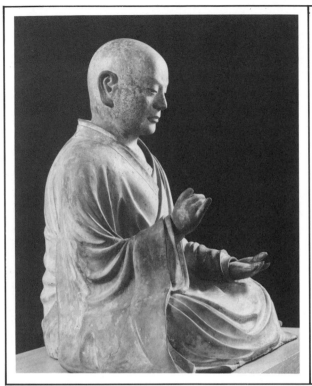

A statue of a Buddhist monk. According to Buddhist philosophy, drinking leads to disease, discord, disturbance of temper, shame, loss of property, and loss of wisdom.

Confucian ethics tend to discourage intoxication, especially in public, and to restrict drinking to mealtime, whether it be a routine supper at home or a lavish banquet. (The Chinese do have a tradition of toasting with high-proof whiskey called *mao tai* during banquets.) And traditional Chinese serve tea, rather than alcohol, to visitors. The Chinese also disapprove of drinking alone and generally try to discourage females and children from drinking. Some Chinese, however, carefully initiate children into the proper, moderate consumption of alcohol.

Traditional Chinese beliefs attribute to alcohol such negative side effects as impairment of intellect and morals, shortening of lifespan, and an increase in criminal behavior. Conversely, moderate alcohol intake is believed to have such benefits as increased blood circulation and blood production and improvement of mental well-being, appetite, and digestion.

Despite the cultural inclination to avoid alcohol abuse, however, the rate of alcoholism appears to be rising among the Chinese — at least among those Chinese living in Hong

Kong and elsewhere who are exposed to Western drinking habits and beverages. Alcohol abuse also occurs in mainland China. In 1987, the Chinese government dispatched about 200 doctors to treat victims of a toxic moonshine liquor that was consumed by people around Naning, the Guangxi province capital about 1,400 miles south of Beijing, the nation's capital.

Buddhist Abstinence in Japan

Like China, Japan has seen times of both acceptance and prohibition of alcohol consumption. With the ascendancy of Buddhist philosophy in Japan in the sixth century C.E., prohibition was decreed from time to time over the next several hundred years. According to Buddhism, drinking led to loss of property, disease, discord, shame, disturbance of temper, and a loss of wisdom.

From 1603 to 1867, laws to decrease production of sake (rice wine) were strongly enforced. Many feudal lords established prohibition on their estates, and some leading scholars advocated or required abstinence among their followers. By the late 19th century, however, Western liquor and drinking customs appeared in Japan, as did the Yokohama Temperance Society, the Hokkaido Temperance Society, and a Japanese branch of the Women's Christian Temperance Union, according to *Beliefs, Behaviors, and Alcoholic Beverages.*

Despite the concern over alcohol abuse, the Japanese have developed a number of drinking customs that require consumption of sake. For example, the *toso* custom, which was introduced from China more than a thousand years ago as a medicinal ritual, required medicines to be mixed with sake on New Year's Day and consumed to prevent disease. Today, ordinary sake is offered to people who visit friends on New Year's Day. Romantic parties are held in August and September to view the full moon while listening to poetry and drinking sake, and both the bride and bridegroom consume sake at Shinto weddings to solemnize the ceremony. Traditionally, younger women did not usually drink alcohol; they were more likely expected to minister to the needs of their inebriated husbands.

After World War II, during which alcohol was rationed, the influx of Western alcoholic beverages combined with several other factors to increase the consumption of alcoholic beverages in Japan. The other contributing factors included the opening of many cabarets and nightclubs in major cities, the establishment of large numbers of beer halls to serve American and British troops, and the introduction of cocktail parties held for the reception of Western residents and visitors. In 1961, a law was passed prohibiting public drunkenness and establishing the first alcoholism treatment center in Japan.

In the 1960s, as Japan became a major world economic power, young Japanese businessmen began consuming more alcoholic beverages, partly to satisfy the expectation that they would socialize with members of their firm after work. An increase in personal freedom, as well as a loosening of the traditionally close families that might have offered guidance, also encouraged new patterns of alcohol consumption. Drinking among Japanese women gradually increased, too, as did the rate of divorce.

Today sake, the traditional alcoholic drink, is losing popularity in Japan. Shochu, a cheaper, generally less-alcoholic distilled spirit similar to vodka and made from barley, corn, or buckwheat, is rapidly becoming a favorite drink.

In prewar Japan, toleration of drunkenness was confined to specific rituals, ceremonies, and recreational gatherings. By defining where and when drunkenness was permitted, this limited permissive attitude acted as a social control of drinking. The new, more permissive drinking attitudes, however, fail to define the areas in which drunkenness is permitted behavior.

Whereas the traditional pattern of Japanese drinking enhanced the sense of social solidarity while avoiding guilt and ambivalence about drinking, disapproval of drunkenness is now increasing. Moreover, Japan now has one of the highest reported rates of alcoholism in the world, along with France and the United States.

The Marijuana-Oriented Culture of India

Among the historical stories recounted in the four *Vedas* (holy books) of the ancient Aryans who invaded India around 2000 B.C.E. is the tale of how the god Siva brought the marijuana plant down from the Himalayas for the Aryans' enjoy-

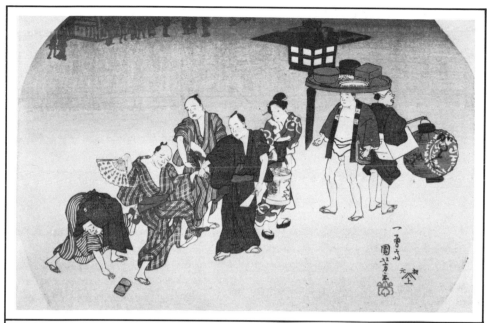

A drunken street scene by the 19th-century Japanese painter Utagawa Kuniyoshi. Sake, the traditional wine made from fermented rice, has long been a part of Japanese rituals and social celebrations.

ment. In his book *Marijuana: The First Twelve Thousand Years* Ernest L. Abel points out that a substance called *bhang*, derived from the dried leaves of the cannabis plant, is cited in the *Vedas* as one of the "five kingdoms of herbs . . . which release us from anxiety."

Bhang is either eaten in the form of small balls or mixed with sugar, milk, and a variety of seeds and spices to produce a drink called *thandai*, according to *Cannabis and Culture*. Because thandai contains nutritious ingredients, such as almonds and milk, it supplements the lower-class diet, which is poor in proteins; the spices supply mineral salts, which are lost in perspiration during the hot summer months.

The drug did not begin to become a part of everyday life in India until the 10th century C.E. However, over the centuries it became so widely used that the Indian Hemp Drugs Commission, established in the 1890s to investigate the use of cannabis in India, concluded that the plant was too integral a part of life in India to curtail its use.

Today, bhang is as common at social and religious gatherings as alcohol is in the United States. The preparation of thandai often occurs in a social atmosphere in which participants discuss issues of the day or family matters.

The exudate of the cannabis plant, called *charas* (from which hashish is derived), and the flowering tops, called ganja, also play an important role in the social lives of people in both villages and cities. Indians mix charas with tobacco to make cigarettes; they smoke ganja in a funnel-shaped clay pipe.

The smoking of ganja (or sometimes even ordinary tobacco) can be an occasion for members of different social classes to intermingle. In order to preserve the ritual purity of the pipe as it is passed around, smokers take puffs from the passage between the right index finger and thumb, rather than directly from the mouthpiece itself.

Because the drug is used only during specific celebrations and ceremonies, and as part of distinct social rituals,

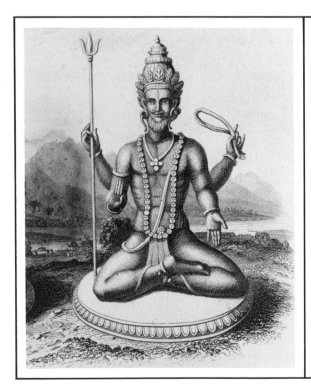

According to the Vedas, sacred texts of Hinduism, the god Siva brought the marijuana plant down from the Himalayas for the Aryans' enjoyment. Today, marijuana use in India is as commonplace as alcohol use in the United States.

the number of regular, heavy users is small, and dependence on cannabis is not common, according to a report on social aspects of cannabis use in India published in *Cannabis and Culture*.

Pakistan Turns From Traditional to Modern Drugs

Pakistan has historically been a major cannabis producer, and various cannabis products have played a traditional role in folk medicine. One concoction, Pakistani *bhang*, is made by boiling cannabis leaves and other ingredients in water.

Interest in hashish was stimulated during the 1960s, when Western youths traveled to the northern areas of Pakistan where hashish was readily available. Today, cannabis abusers are mostly members of the lower socioeconomic groups, particularly in the provinces of Punjab, Sind, and Northwest Frontier Province.

Abuse of psychoactive substances, including methaqualone, is now spreading in Pakistan. In response, the government is expanding treatment facilities and launching preventive education programs. Benzodiazepines are abused by the wealthy and literate portion of the Pakistani population to ward off the tensions of daily life, according to a 1984 report published in *Impact of Science on Society*, by Dr. Inamul Haq, a Pakistani pharmacist with that country's National Institute of Health. The supply is ample, with about 10 brands of benzodiazepines marketed in the country.

Pakistan's Violent Heroin Traffickers

In December 1986, Pakistani police launched a major drug raid in Karachi, a seaport town on the Arabian Sea. Police moved into a suburb populated by a group of Afghan and Pakistani Muslims called Pathans. There, according to official reports, the police seized 600 pounds of heroin in Sohrab Got, a Pathan colony of brick and concrete hovels. However, the drug chieftains were tipped off about the impending raid and escaped.

Following the raid, a group of Pathans waged an organized campaign of terror against non-Pathan neighborhoods. The criminals roamed the streets in jeeps, shooting at people in stores and bus stops and setting fires. The bloody riot, which was aimed at the Pathans' old ethnic enemies, the Mohajirs, was apparently backed by heroin traffickers trying to divert the attention of officials from drug trafficking.

The apparent immunity of Pakistan's drug traffickers to public pressure is similar to the hold that these criminals have in other countries—Colombia, for example.

The opium trafficked out of the slums of Karachi and into the affluent neighborhoods of the city comes from the forests of Pakistan's Northwest Frontier Province. This area is home to a traditionally uncontrollable tribal population that has now been augmented by hundreds of thousands of Afghanistan refugees from the war in that neighboring country.

Despite government efforts to curtail their cultivation of poppies, Pakistani farmers produced more than 10 metric tons of opium in 1986 — probably in response to a growing demand for opium worldwide and a rising market price for it. During the 1970s, the opium was refined in Turkey, Sicily, and elsewhere for the U.S. and European heroin markets. But in the 1980s, laboratories emerged in Pakistan itself. According to the *Department of State Bulletin* for September 1986, like many other countries that serve as centers for the drug trade, Pakistan now suffers from a major outbreak in heroin addiction as a result of the drug trafficking.

Heroin dens, known as *saqi khana*, are often located underground in crowded business areas. Potential customers are lured inside with the offer of free drugs. Some young people try narcotics out of curiosity or after being pressured by peers, and many who become heroin addicts already have a history of multiple drug use.

The majority of heroin addicts belong to the middle or upper-middle class and are between 18 and 25 years old. By 1984, there were about 170,000 heroin addicts in Pakistan. The country now has between 300,000 and 1 million heroin addicts. And according to the Report of the International Narcotics Control Board for 1986, more than half a million Pakistanis are also addicted to opium and cannabis.

According to Dr. Inamul Haq, who described Pakistan's opiate addiction problem in his 1984 report in *Impact of Science on Society*, opium was a traditional medicine in the Indo-Pakistan area for many centuries, where it was used as

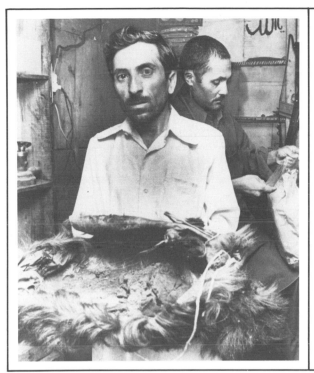

A drug merchant displays his wares in the Bara market in the Northwest Frontier Province in Pakistan. Although hashish use was once widespread in Pakistan, it has now been replaced by use of more dangerous drugs such as heroin, opium, and methaqualone.

a sedative. Today, there are tens of thousands of practitioners of alternate systems of medicine, such as homeopathy, many of whom use opium to treat insomnia, diarrhea, dysentery, diabetes, rheumatism, cough, and digestive troubles in children. In fact, some uneducated mothers give opium to children who suffer teething problems. Nevertheless, the majority of opium addicts are found among people 50 to 60 years old in the lower economic strata of society.

Opium, heroin, cannabis, and methaqualone are abused in Afghanistan as well, and the government there is developing prevention, treatment, and rehabilitation programs to cope with the problem.

The *Department of State Bulletin* also reported in 1986 that despite denials from the governments of Afghanistan and Iran, illicit opium production is not controlled in those countries. Moreover, there is evidence that Iran has a huge heroin-addict population and might be a net importer of opium from Afghanistan and Pakistan despite export of opium from Iran's northwestern areas. In addition, opiates produced in Afghanistan and bound for Western markets are transshipped through Iran.

Marijuana's Long History in Southeast Asia

Cannabis indica, the marijuana plant grown in Southeast Asia, has the highest content of Delta-9 THC, the active ingredient of marijuana, of all the cannabis species.

According to *Cannabis and Culture*, the plant was probably introduced into Cambodia (now called Kampuchea), Laos, Thailand, and Vietnam, around the 16th century, and became integrated into the cuisine, medical beliefs, and social customs of the area.

Distrust of the drug does exist among individuals whose cultural and social attitudes have come to resemble those of Western countries. The peasants, however, usually grow the plant around their houses. The leaves and stalks add a euphoric quality and flavor to food; many peasants use it to combat illnesses, coughing, and nervousness, and to facilitate digestion and childbirth. As in some other cultures, such as the khat chewers in Africa and ganja smokers in Jamaica, marijuana eases the burdens of the workday and facilitates social interaction. Thus, regular cannabis use is not generally considered to be wrong, although smokers who consume vast quantities of marijuana regularly become habituated and suffer when deprived of the drug.

Marijuana's Move from Culture to Crime

By the 1980s, marijuana was no longer just a cultural phenomenon in Southeast Asia. Marijuana crop destruction programs carried out by officials in Mexico and parts of South America threatened the supply of major drug traffickers. In response, American traffickers turned Thailand's poor farmers into suppliers of high-grade marijuana. Working through Thai middlemen, the traffickers began to supply farmers with seed, fertilizer, and insecticides.

Marijuana grows easily in the vast wastelands and uninhabited regions of Thailand, and many poor farmers welcomed the opportunity to receive a steady income from this illegal crop, whose high quality commands a premium price in the United States and Australia.

Nurtured by the lure of money, marijuana farming spread across the Thai border into Laos, one of the world's poorest countries, with a population of 3.6 million.

In 1987, the *New York Times* quoted the head of the Thai National Security Council as saying that a Laotian government agency was buying marijuana seed and fertilizer in Thailand, distributing it in Laos, and purchasing the subsequent crop from local farmers for resale abroad. The Laotian government has denied this accusation, although Thai officials claimed that Laos exported at least 200 tons of marijuana in the first half of 1987.

China Loses Opium Wars and Gains Addicts

Rows of half-conscious men lying on slabs in a dimly lit room puffing opium pipes: This is one of the darker images of China. It is believed that Dutch traders introduced opium to China in the 17th century. The Chinese used the imported drug mostly as a medicine, to relieve pain, and did not at first cultivate the opium poppy.

By the 1830s, greedy merchants with Britain's East India Company, as well as traders from Portugal, France, and Amer-

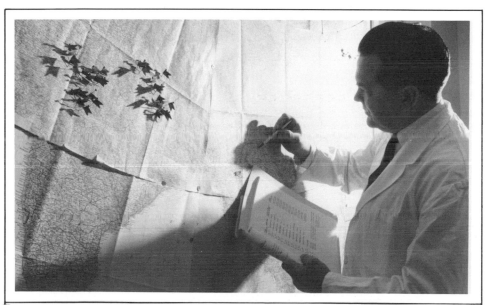

Dr. Olav Braenden of the UN Laboratory in Geneva points to the major opium-producing areas. Much of the heroin in the United States is grown in the Golden Triangle countries of Laos, Burma, and Thailand.

ica, were illegally importing thousands of chests of opium into China each year. Eventually, feudal Chinese landlords compelled their peasants to cultivate opium, as well.

The opium business turned countless Chinese into addicts and drained the Chinese economy, as huge sums of money were poured into opium production and importation. When the use of opium threatened to turn into a major social and monetary disaster, the Chinese emperor ordered opium trafficking stopped and supplies burned. The Western traffickers were outraged. Tensions rose to the boiling point between China and the European countries, especially France and Britain. Between 1839 and 1860, a series of bloody conflicts called the Opium Wars brought China to its knees.

The Opium Wars pitted primitive Chinese crossbows against European muskets. Defeated, China was forced to pay millions of dollars to the victors, cede Hong Kong to the British, and continue to receive opium. Thus, Western traders forcefully wove opium into the fabric of Chinese society, leaving the problem behind long after that country was free of their domination.

Following World War II and the establishment of the People's Republic of China, the Chinese government embarked on a major effort to end the cultivation, processing, and trafficking of narcotic drugs. Harsh antidrug laws were put into effect to discourage both Chinese and foreign smugglers. Nevertheless, smuggling continued into the 1980s, with traffickers disguised as tourists bringing the drug into the country by jumbo jets rather than trading ships.

British Hong Kong Inherits the Habit

Britain took possession of Hong Kong from China during the Opium Wars and used this tiny colony off the southeast coast of China as a center for its opium trade with that country. Toward the end of the 19th century, supplies were also exported to the United States. As with South American countries involved in the trafficking of cocaine, the opium trade in Hong Kong soon created a large population of users. Not until 1959 were stringent efforts made to enforce the law against opium use in Hong Kong. By then, abuse was widespread.

Today, opiate abuse in the form of heroin addiction appears to have stabilized in Hong Kong, which has about

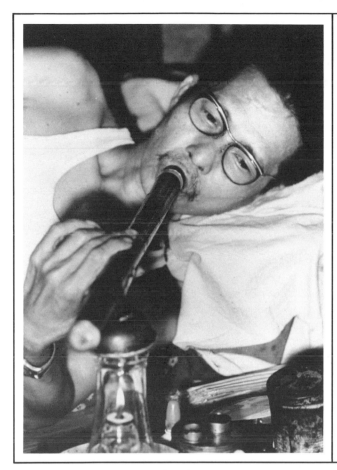

A Laotian man smokes opium in a pipe. Although the medicinal use of narcotics is beneficial, the abuse of those same drugs can be addictive and deadly.

50,000 addicts out of a population of about 5.5 million. Perhaps as a cultural remnant of the opium dens of China, Hong Kong addicts use a smokable heroin. Injectable heroin continues to be shipped from Hong Kong to the United States, as well as to Europe, Canada, and Australia, despite efforts of law-enforcement officials and substantial seizures of drugs.

The Golden Triangle

The Golden Triangle — a region of Southeast Asia where Burma, Laos, and Thailand intersect — is one of the major sources of the heroin sold in the United States. The legal governments of the three countries that merge in the Triangle lack control over the outlying mountain areas where opium is grown. In fact, these areas are home to ethnic tribes and rebel movements, some of which have their own private armies. Opium provides local warlords with a far greater source of cash than any other crop could. Frequently, the warlords have fought among themselves for control of the trade.

An opium warlord named Khun Sa, who supports an armed rebellion against Burma from his heavily fortified strongholds along the Burma-Thailand border, has currently gained control and continues to supply the drug to smugglers despite the military efforts of both countries.

The Burmese government has had some success against other rebel armies involved in opium smuggling. And in Thailand the United Nations' crop substitution program has helped to end farmers' dependence on the opium poppy as a cash crop.

Other programs are now under way to treat addicts and reduce the population of opium users in Southeast Asia. In Thailand, for example, thousands of people have received treatment in Buddhist temples, where priests treat patients with traditional folk medicine. Some Thai addicts even become priests as a way to escape their lives of addiction, according to a 1984 report in *Impact of Science on Society.* Moreover, in Bangkok, Thailand, which still has many opium dens, the effort to dissuade poor, unemployed young people from using drugs includes a program to encourage them to take up breeding locally popular exotic fish for export.

The ethnic group in Laos called the Hmong have traditionally used opium for both social and medical reasons, and Hmong refugees to the United States brought this custom with them to Minnesota. The St. Paul *Pioneer Press-Dispatch* reported in 1986 that about 200 of the 15,000 refugees in that city were opium addicts. The occasional parcel of opium that arrived from Asia in previous years has been replaced with a steady supply from Mexico.

Most of the addicts are men in their 30s and 40s, unemployed and having trouble adjusting to American life. Like many addicts in Southeast Asia, the American immigrants' addiction drains their families' resources. Many of the St. Paul Hmong families have experienced malnourishment.

The government of Laos, however, has done little to prevent or treat opium addiction. On the contrary, there have been reports that it may actually encourage if not subsidize opium production.

Both Thailand and Burma have instituted programs to intercept acetic anhydride, a chemical used to convert opium to heroin. As a result, traffickers have shifted laboratories south — near the border of Malaysia, a country with a large number of drug addicts and a particularly harsh antidrug enforcement program. The death penalty is mandatory if a drug offender is caught carrying more than 15 grams of heroin, which is considered proof of trafficking. Two young Australians arrested in 1983 for drug trafficking in Malaysia were hanged three years later. A few hours after that, a 69-year-old Malaysian woman was sentenced to death for dealing in heroin.

The number of newly reported heroin addicts has declined in Malaysia, perhaps because of the government's harsh stand on heroin trafficking and its efforts at rehabilitation. Nevertheless, heroin continues to be smuggled into the country, or produced there in conversion laboratories, either for local consumption or transport to Australia and Europe.

Other drugs abused in Southeast Asia include the psychotropic drug methaqualone in Burma and amphetamine in Thailand. The stringent antiheroin measures in Malaysia have decreased the availability of that drug, but encourage the use of psychotropic substances as substitutes.

Japan's Cycle of Drug Abuse

Stimulant abuse has a long history among the hard-working, ambitious population of Japan. Before World War II, laborers used such drugs to help them complete their tasks, as did some university professors trying to keep up with demanding schedules. During the war, amphetamines were given to factory workers, army troops, and *kamikaze* pilots who flew suicide missions against American warships in the Pacific. After the war, stockpiled drugs made their way onto the black market.

When the government began to crack down on the black market in 1951, organized crime took over the task of production and distribution. Police responded harshly, arresting more than 55,000 people for drug offenses in 1954, when the number of drug users was estimated at 550,000. By the late 1950s, amphetamine abuse was greatly reduced from earlier years, and gangsters turned to heroin trafficking. But

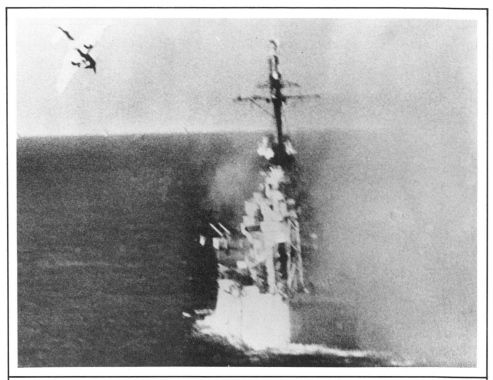

During World War II amphetamines were given to Japanese factory workers and army troops to treat fatigue. Kamikaze pilots were also given amphetamines before they flew their suicide missions.

by the mid-1960s, police had swept Japan clean of most of the major dealers, and the heroin problem subsided.

In the affluent days of the 1970s, during which Japan emerged on the world scene as a major economic power, heroin dealers released from prison began setting up amphetamine distribution networks, according to a 1987 report in the *Christian Science Monitor*. The drugs, imported illegally from South Korea and Taiwan, fed the new demand among hard-working housewives and students as well as traditional users such as truck drivers and other laborers.

Amphetamines and, to some extent, paint thinner (which is sniffed) are the major drugs of abuse in Japan today. There is also heavy consumption of sleeping pills and barbiturates in Japan. The country's island geography and tight police security virtually exclude drugs that must be imported, such as cocaine and marijuana, according to a 1986 report in the San Jose *Mercury News*.

The newspaper also reported that officials estimate there are now hundreds of thousands of Japanese addicts in this nation of 120 million people. Yet as of 1986, there was only one treatment facility.

Amphetamine trafficking produces about half the income of the Yakuza, Japan's organized crime group. Indeed, drug addicts themselves are widely viewed as criminals, and there is insufficient sympathy in the government to expend tax money on treatment facilities.

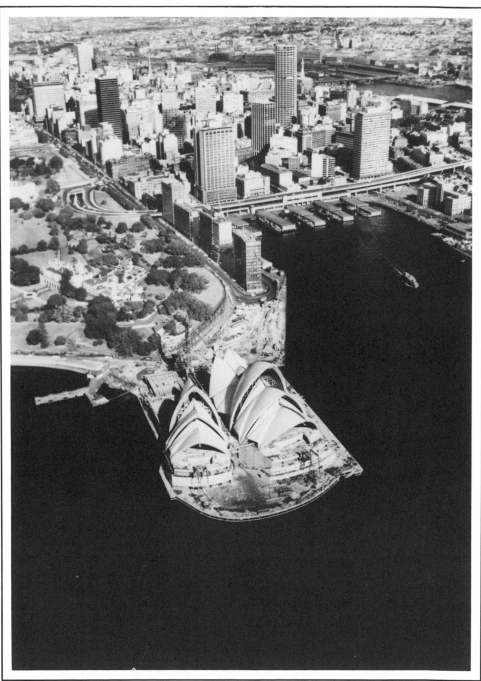

Sydney is the oldest city in Australia. In recent years, the city has undergone a dramatic transformation, counting among its recent additions gleaming new skyscrapers and a growing drug abuse problem.

CHAPTER 8

USE AND ABUSE IN AUSTRALIA, NEW ZEALAND, AND POLYNESIA

During the 18th century, when Australia was used as a British prison colony, liquor was deemed so important there that it was used as a medium of exchange in place of money. It was also a defense against loneliness, desperation, and despair — among male and female convicts as well as among free men and women.

Convict life was often brutal at penal colonies, such as the camp at Port Macquarie, New South Wales, where physically disabled workers struggled alongside the insane to complete assigned tasks and survive another day. Rum aided life in that colony, as Robert Hughes points out in his book about the founding of Australia, *The Fatal Shore*.

Hughes describes how the "men on timber," those with wooden legs, when not otherwise employed "... would lie sunning themselves and gazing at the sea, guzzling rum, of which there was plenty at Port Macquarie, cooked up in illicit convict stills from the sugar cane that flourished there. Real men drank it laced with tobacco juice, a mixture believed to kill the pain of flogging."

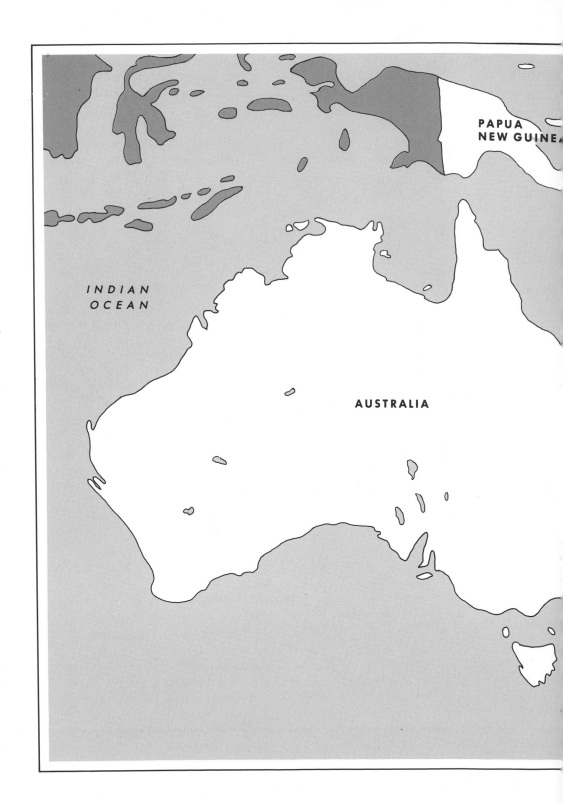

PAPUA
NEW GUINEA

INDIAN
OCEAN

AUSTRALIA

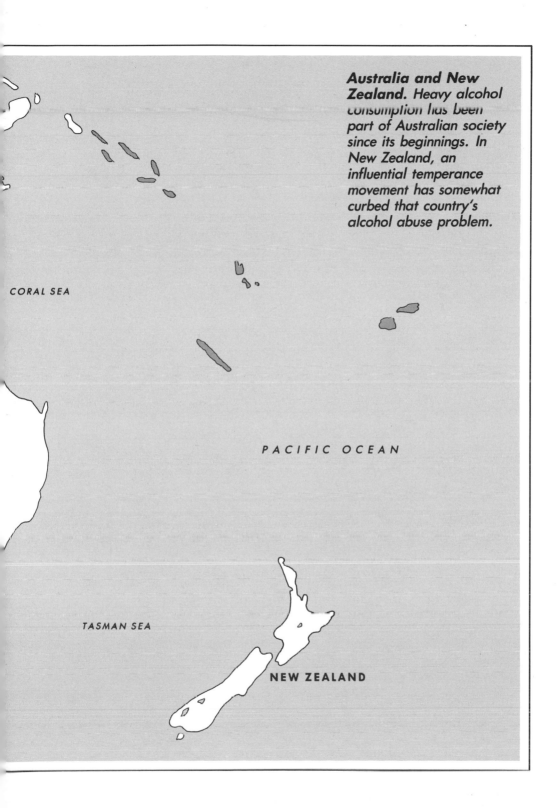

Australia and New Zealand. Heavy alcohol consumption has been part of Australian society since its beginnings. In New Zealand, an influential temperance movement has somewhat curbed that country's alcohol abuse problem.

CORAL SEA

PACIFIC OCEAN

TASMAN SEA

NEW ZEALAND

Aborigines Switch from Hallucinogens to Alcohol

Rum, so popular in the white society, contributed to the demise of the culture of the aborigines. These black native residents of Australia lost their land and their lives when marauding whites, with their sheep and cattle, pushed the aborigines off their ancestral hunting grounds, numbed them with liquor, and butchered them.

Before the encroachment of the white colonists, the aborigine tribes had well-established cultures that included the use of the *pituri* plant (*Duboisia hopwoodii*), according to *Hallucinogens: Cross-Cultural Perspectives*. The plant contains the alkaloids scopolamine and hyoscyamine, which produce hallucinations when ingested. The aborigines consumed pituri to quell hunger and thirst during their long travels in the desert. They also offered the plant to each other as a token of friendship and chewed it in order to facilitate social interaction. Extensive trade routes, called pituri roads, enabled the aborigines to travel far and wide, trading the pituri plant with other tribes for spears, boomerangs, nets, shields, fish, and yams.

But the coming of the whites changed the aborigine way of life. Some were isolated on reserves, much as American Indians were placed on reservations in the 19th century. Like American Indians, many of these aborigines succumbed to Western diseases, such as smallpox, and others became alcoholics.

By 1840, for example, the town of Brisbane, formerly economically and socially dominated by its penal colony, had made the transition to an independent community. "And the broken, marginal Aborigines," wrote Hughes in *The Fatal Shore,* "stupefied with cane liquor, dozing like lumps of shadow in patches of shade, confirmed the total victory of white civilization."

Bars and Bloodhouses

In the traditionally male-dominated Australian society, women were virtually excluded from bars and taverns, which were crowded with shouting, boisterous men downing beers. Women were relegated to drab lounges at the back of the pubs. Today, however, women freely patronize drinking es-

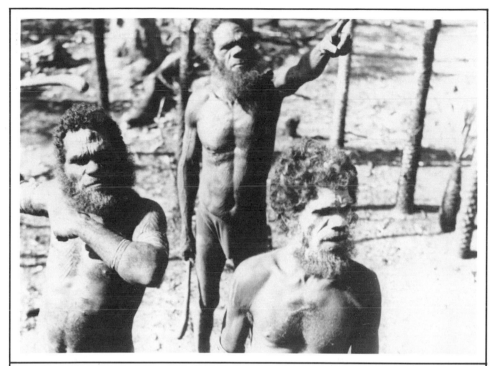

Before the encroachment of the white settlers, the aborigines, the native inhabitants of Australia, were a well established culture that used the hallucinogenic plant pituri *to quell hunger on long journeys.*

tablishments — except for the few "bloodhouses" that still cater to a rowdy, men-only crowd.

Alcohol, then, has played an integral part in the cultural history of Australia since its very beginnings, although the drink of choice is now beer, rather than rum. Indeed, the country's 1980 average of 38 gallons for every man, woman, and child put it in third place, behind Germany and Czechoslovakia, in beer consumption.

During the 1980s, however, many drinkers switched to low-alcohol beer, perhaps in response to the introduction of random blood-alcohol tests, which police began to give motorists. Australia's scattered population is connected by about a million miles of roads, many of which are unpaved. Drunk drivers have contributed greatly to accidents on Australia's rugged highways, where death rates are twice as high as Great Britain's.

From 1978 to 1985, per capita consumption of beer fell by 10%, during which time the country's economy was less prosperous than during the 30 years following World War II, according to a 1987 report in the *Medical Journal of Australia*. The aging of Australia's population also appears to have contributed to the decrease in consumption. Nevertheless, the country's overall rate of alcohol consumption remains the 11th highest in the world, exceeding that of New Zealand (15th) by 8%, of the United States (18th) by 24%, and of the United Kingdom (23rd) by 50%.

Over the past few decades, concern about alcohol-related accidents and medical problems has prompted an increase in research on the issue and the establishment in 1981 of the Australian Medical Society on Alcohol and Drug Related Problems. Special university and medical-school courses now address the problem, and a biannual journal, *Australian Alcohol/Drug Review*, publishes scientific articles on the subject.

Even as health authorities labor to contain the alcohol problem, Australian wines, which have gained an interna-

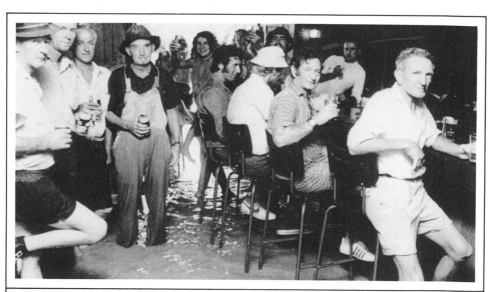

Workers in Sydney brave a torrential rainstorm complete with flooding at a neighborhood bar. In response to growing concern over alcohol consumption, many Australians have switched to low-alcohol beer.

tional reputation for quality, are becoming extremely popular. The burgeoning interest in wine is reflected in the reports of wine columnists in Australian newspapers and in the wine supplements, guides, and advertising in magazines.

Australian Drinking Starts Early

The high rate of alcohol consumption is also reflected in the drinking habits of the youth of Australia. In 1987, the *Medical Journal of Australia* reported that a national survey of more than 23,000 school children aged 12 to 17 showed that 97% of the 16 year olds had tried alcohol. At age 12, 23% of boys and 14% of girls had reported that they had drunk alcohol in the past week. Those figures rose to 56% of boys and 49% of girls by age 17.

Moreover, the *International Journal of the Addictions* reported in 1985 that alcohol is the most frequently used drug among Australian youths. Other substances, in order of their frequency of use, include tobacco, painkillers, cannabis, barbiturates, inhalants, and amphetamines. Opiates, cocaine, and hallucinogens were not in widespread use.

Australia Fights Its Other Drug Problems

Heroin abuse among the population as a whole is a problem, however, and illegally produced amphetamines are widely available, despite the destruction of several clandestine laboratories in the past few years.

In 1986, Australian prime minister Bob Hawke and the state premiers launched a three-year campaign to fight drug abuse through education, rehabilitation, and law enforcement. The rehabilitation measures included extra funding for methadone programs, detoxification units, halfway houses, and community-based agencies.

Alcohol Control and Prohibition in New Zealand

European colonizers and traders brought alcohol to New Zealand during the 19th century. Following a period of heavy alcohol use, which caused widespread social problems including public drunkenness, an influential temperance movement led to prohibition in many localities.

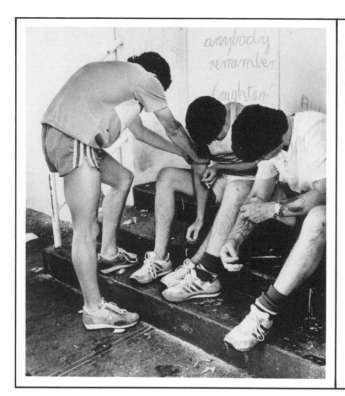

Young Australian junkies shoot up with heroin. Australia is now facing a growing heroin abuse problem.

From 1920 to 1940, the prohibition movement gradually lost ground. But the alcohol-consuming public was dissatisfied with the inadequate distribution of drinking establishments around the country and the shabby condition of many of those that existed. There was little incentive for owners to fix up their businesses, and often, little money with which to do so. Meanwhile, an increasing number of "dry" districts voted to restore drinking.

In response, New Zealand passed the 1949 Licensing Trust Act, which offered individual districts the option of establishing publicly funded, board-run, acceptable drinking establishments. Under the Act, private individuals can apply for licenses in the area controlled by the trust, but local trusts have a preferential right to the initial hotel or tavern license in the area. Public boards distribute a portion of the profits they make in the form of grants, loans, and donations to the local community.

For the next few decades after the act was passed, alcohol consumption rose dramatically, as did alcohol-related problems. The government responded in 1976 by establishing the

Alcoholic Liquor Advisory Council, which is active in supporting treatment facilities and advising the government on policy and education.

Public support for restrictions on alcohol is not likely to come from the influential middle class, which includes lawmakers and members of the communications industry (which receives considerable revenue from liquor advertising). This group, as a whole, is most likely to have a liberal attitude toward personal use of alcohol, according to a 1985 report in the *British Journal of Addiction*. Moreover, this group is increasingly supportive of New Zealand's burgeoning wine industry, which, as in the case of Australia's wine industry, is attracting many consumers.

Isolation Does Not Stop Drug Abuse

New Zealand's geographical isolation limits the availability of illicit drugs. Nevertheless, some heroin enters the country from Australia, and LSD arrives by mail from the Netherlands,

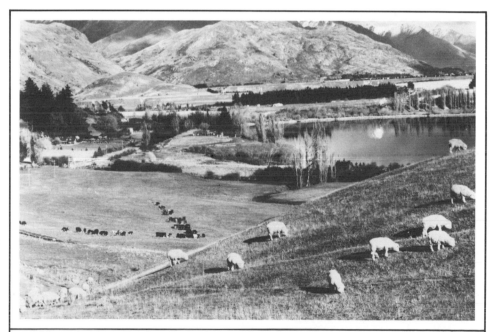

Although New Zealand's isolation does limit the number of illicit drugs that are available there, both heroin and LSD are smuggled in.

according to the United Nations' 1986 report of the International Narcotics Control Board.

In addition, there is illicit manufacture of morphine and heroin from both legally and illegally obtained preparations containing codeine. Cannabis oil is extracted domestically, mostly from locally cultivated cannabis. Authorities have also seized cocaine, some of which might have been destined for Australia.

Kava: Polynesia's Original Drink of Choice

Before white traders first came ashore to sample the delights of the South Pacific islands in the mid-18th century, Polynesian natives, like most of the Indians of North America, had no alcoholic beverages. Instead, residents of many of these islands prepared a drink called *kava* from the roots of *Piper methysticum*, a member of the pepper family.

The drink, still consumed in some areas of the South Pacific, does not produce hallucinations. Rather, the concoction induces a state of mild intoxication, often accompanied by a pleasant state of relaxation that may eventually lead to sleep. Its active ingredient, dihydromethysticin, is similar to these substances that produce nutmeg intoxication.

Consumption of kava was widespread among natives of Fiji and other South Pacific islands before the coming of white traders and missionaries during the late 18th and early 19th centuries. Kava ceremonies were customarily limited to men, who sat cross-legged in a circle and shared the drink from a common cup. The ingestion of kava was usually accompanied by a rite performed by chiefs and priests, and in western Polynesia — especially Samoa and Tonga — it became a sacred ceremony. According to a report in *Beliefs, Behaviors, and Alcoholic Beverages*, the ceremony distinguished titled from untitled persons and symbolically validated status differences between chiefs.

Drinking Customs Replace Kava Customs

In the mid-1800s, white traders and escaped convicts from the Australian continent helped spread the technique of distilling alcoholic beverages throughout the South Pacific. Tahitians, who learned to make a crude wine called "bush beer" from orange juice, brought the technique to the Cook Islands, much to the dismay of Christian missionaries who were trying to "civilize" the natives. Consumption of alcoholic beverages in the Cook Islands, especially on the islands of Atiu, Rortonga, and Aitutaki, became highly ritualized, resembling, in that respect, the kava ceremony. On these islands, drinking sessions are under the control of a leader, called a *tuati*, who remains sober. Drinkers sing hymns and carry on discussions about sex, farming, politics, and other important matters under the watchful eye of the tuati, who ejects disruptive drinkers. It is believed that the drinking group maintains continuity with older cultural values and helps to preserve social organization.

Polynesians in the Society Islands, especially Tahiti, retain a somewhat festive attitude toward drinking that developed during the 19th century. However, with the coming of

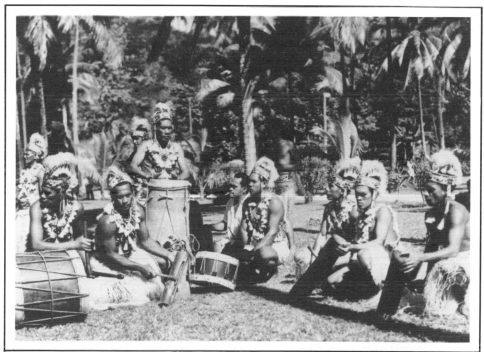

Tahitian men prepare for a feast day. The consumption of kava and other intoxicating beverages made from local plants or fruit often accompanies feast days and other social celebrations on the South Pacific islands.

the French, a blight on the orange groves, and the deaths of the foremost native brewmasters in the early 20th century, Tahitians turned to wine and beer.

Weekend drinking became commonplace as the European traditions of regular workweeks and a money economy influenced life on the Society Islands. Nevertheless, festive native drinking bouts recur from time to time. Society Islanders prefer beverages of low alcoholic content, such as beer, which help them to achieve a physical and psychic state associated with their singing and dancing — without making them groggy.

Tahitian men are generally quiet and shy and often use alcohol to facilitate their sexual approaches to women. Drinking does sometimes lead to fighting among Tahitians, although the aggression is mostly verbal or limited to random pushing and slapping. Tahitian women also drink, and they, too, occasionally fight when drunk.

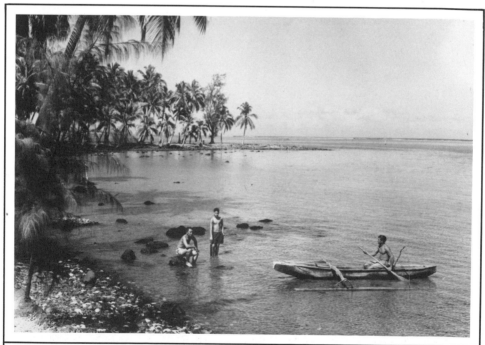

Tahitians' preference for low-alcohol beverages and slow drinking reflects their health-conscious attitude. In fact, organized sporting events have helped to decrease alcohol consumption in some areas.

Overall, drinking fits into the Tahitian value system of collective eating, singing, dancing, and sexual communion. The preference for low-alcohol beverages and slow drinking appears to reflect their health-conscious attitude. Indeed, organized sports programs have been instrumental in decreasing drinking in some areas.

Unlike Tahitian drinking, Samoan consumption of alcohol is not ritualized nor is it based on village- or district-wide festive behavior. Nor is the aggression it provokes as harmless as it is on Tahiti.

Most Samoans learned about brewing and drinking from New Zealand troops during World War I and from American troops during World War II. The Samoans' high-alcohol content brew, called *fa'amafu*, is made from imported malt, hops, sugar, and yeast, rather than from native fruit. Drinking groups consist mostly of males, some younger than 15.

Samoan society emphasizes conformity, acceptance of group decisions, ceremonial compliance, and politeness. Aggression and disagreement tend to be suppressed, surfacing only with intoxication. Young, titled men, especially, shoulder the burden of silent conformity and respect, and it is these men who most often display the drunken aggressiveness that sometimes leads to injury or even death.

The Betel Nut and Booze on the Admiralties

Natives of the Admiralty Islands, now part of Papua New Guinea, also had no knowledge of alcohol before the arrival of Europeans in the 19th century. Kava ceremonies were restricted to a few islands of this group. But residents of the Admiralties and of southern Asia in general have for centuries chewed a stimulant concoction made from betel palm seeds (betel nuts) smeared onto a betel pepper leaf (*Piper betel*), together with aromatic flavorings and lime paste. The betel nut is still used to promote wakefulness and stamina, despite the inroads alcohol has made into drug-consuming customs.

In 1962, the prohibition of the sale of alcoholic beverages to natives was replaced by an antidiscrimination law that permitted natives to purchase and consume beer. The next year, the law was modified to include any alcoholic beverage. This pleased the natives, many of whom felt that to emulate the Europeans who drank alcohol was to gain prestige.

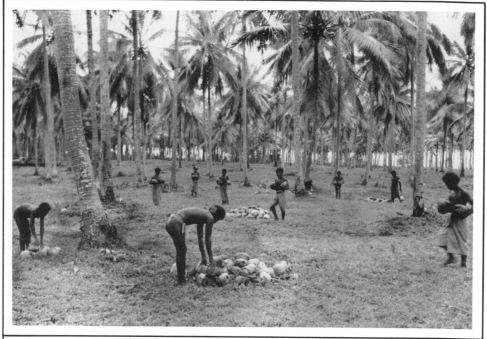

Natives on the islands of Micronesia gather coconuts to manufacture a home-grown alcoholic drink distilled from fermented coconut oil.

The Battle for Souls in Micronesia

American whaling ships plying the waters of the South Pacific during the first half of the 19th century found the Marshall, Caroline, and Gilbert island groups in Micronesia to be ideal ports of call. Several individual islands in the groups, especially Guam, Kusaie, and Ponape, offered the sailors food, water, wood, and an idyllic place to stretch their legs.

When American missionaries arrived in the 18th and 19th centuries, they found beach communities of sailors who did little more than drink, chase island women, and fight. The natives, introduced to alcoholic beverages and technology, were manufacturing and consuming rum, as well as a home-grown alcoholic drink distilled from fermented coconut oil. The Micronesians not only drank liquor but actively sought it out, and they traded almost anything of value to get it.

Although the missionaries used alcohol abstinence as a measure to separate Christians from heathens, kava consumption, which existed in Micronesia only on the islands of Kusaie and Ponape, was singled out on those islands because of its importance in native religions. The missionaries managed to stop kava ceremonies for good on Kusaie, but the tradition has persisted on Ponape. The conflicting attitudes toward liquor learned by the Micronesians are reflected to this day — especially in eastern Micronesia — by the ambivalence of the natives toward this drug.

Although alcohol abuse occurs throughout Polynesia, the general desire for psychic rapport with others tends to minimize the extent of the destructive use of the drug. Destructive drinking isolates the abuser from friends and family, a situation not desired in Polynesia.

In some areas, natives shy away from alcohol consumption and turn toward more traditional means of socializing. For instance, the communal practice of kava drinking has undergone a revival in Samoa and other Polynesian islands, apparently reflecting a rising resentment among the natives toward white intrusion into their cultures.

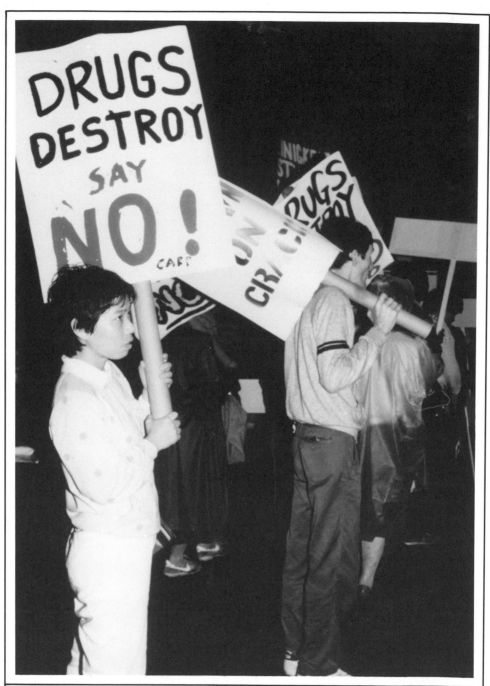

An antidrug demonstration in front of the United Nations. In the past, drugs played an important role in both religious and social celebrations. Today their abuse is a worldwide threat.

CHAPTER 9

CONCLUSION

In most ancient cultures, drug abuse was limited to a few errant fellows who overindulged after a hard day's labor or to the town drunkard consuming too much mead. But in the modern age, increased sophistication has brought with it techniques of drug production and distribution that have resulted in a worldwide epidemic of abuse.

What began in the past as drug *use* — stimulants and intoxicants employed in carefully structured religious ceremonies or social celebrations — has today evolved into drug *abuse*. Each year, tens of thousands of people die as a result of their experimentation with drugs. Many more are murdered either by those under the influence or for standing in the way of the criminals who run the drug underworld.

Looking to the past, to the history of drug use in ancient cultures throughout the world, may not give us any answers to cure the problems that face us today. However, tracing the path of drug usage in a culture can give us insight into the problem. It can, perhaps, tell us something about the different needs of the people involved and of the upheavals in modern society that foster a dependency on mind-altering substances. And it may give us clues as to the most effective methods of treating drug abusers in various cultures.

Further Reading

Abel, Ernest L. *Marijuana: The First Twelve Thousand Years*. New York: McGraw Hill, 1982.

De Rios, Marlene. *Hallucinogens: Cross-Cultural Perspectives*. Albuquerque: University of New Mexico Press, 1984.

Dolan, Edward., Jr. *International Drug Traffic*. New York: Franklin Watts, 1985.

Everett, Michael W., Jack O. Waddell, and Dwight B. Heath, eds. *Cross-Cultural Approaches to the Study of Alcohol*. The Hague: Mouton Publishers, 1973.

Goodwin, Donald W. *Alcoholism: The Facts*. New York: Oxford University Press, 1981.

Grinspoon, Lester, and James B. Bakalar. *Psychedelic Drugs Reconsidered*. New York: Basic Books, 1979.

Illegal Drugs and Alcohol: America's Anguish. Plano, TX: Information Aids, 1985.

International Narcotics Control Strategy Report, 1987. Bureau of International Narcotics Matters, U.S. Department of State, 1987.

Kirsch, M. M. *Designer Drugs*. Minneapolis, MN: Comp-Care, 1986.

McCoy, Alfred W. *The Politics of Heroin in Southeast Asia*. New York: Harper & Row, 1972.

Phillips, Joel L., and Ronald D. Wynne. *Cocaine: The Mystique and the Reality*. New York: Avon Books, 1980.

Marshall, Mac, ed. *Beliefs, Behaviors & Alcoholic Beverages: A Cross-Cultural Survey*. Ann Arbor: University of Michigan Press, 1974.

Report of the International Narcotics Control Board for 1986. Vienna: United Nations Publication, 1986.

Rubin, V., ed. *Cannabis and Culture*. The Hague: Mouton Publishers, 1974.

Glossary

Acquired Immune Deficiency Syndrome (AIDS); a weakening of the body's immune system caused by a virus (HIV); thought to be transmitted through the blood or body secretions during sexual intercourse, transfusions, or the sharing of syringes

addiction a condition caused by repeated drug use, characterized by a compulsive urge to continue using the drug, a tendency to increase the dosage, and physiological and/or psychological dependence

alcoholism alcohol abuse causing deterioration in health and social relations

amphetamine a drug that stimulates the central nervous system, alleviates fatigue, and produces a feeling of alertness and well-being. Although it has been used for weight control, repeated use of the drug can cause restlessness and insomnia

barbiturate a drug that causes depression of the central nervous system and respiration. The drug has toxic side effects and, when used excessively, can lead to tolerance, dependence, and even death

bazuco a cigarette containing both cocaine and tobacco along with dangerously large quantities of kerosene, gasoline, ether, and other chemicals used to transform coca leaves into coca paste. Found primarily in Colombia, bazuco gives a quick, intense high, followed by a craving for more of the drug

bhang a drug used in India and derived from the dried leaves of the cannabis plant; usually eaten in small balls or mixed with milk, sugar, and a variety of seeds and spices to produce a drink called thandai

chica a native fermented beer, considered to be a traditional drink throughout much of Latin America. Chica, or "maize beer," was a staple commodity throughout the Inca Empire

cirrhosis a chronic disease of the liver caused by alcohol poisoning; results in the loss of functioning liver cells and increased resistance to blood flow through the liver

cocaine the primary psychoactive ingredient in the coca plant and a behavioral stimulant

cokomoe the Bahamian name for crack

crack a crude, relatively inexpensive, highly addictive form of cocaine

designer drug a synthetic drug produced by chemically altering the structure of the original, often illicit, drug; a drug that has been redesigned to increase appeal. Crack is a redesigned form of cocaine

fentanyl a synthetic drug with effects similar to those of morphine, but more potent

ganja the Jamaican word for marijuana; ganja is a major component of the Rastafarian life-style and is often smoked or drunk as a tea

hallucinogen a drug that produces sensory impressions that have no basis in reality

hashish a psychoactive substance made from the dried and pressed flowers and leaves of the hemp plant; it contains a high concentration of THC, the active ingredient in the plant

heroin a semisynthetic opiate produced by a chemical modification of morphine

homeopathy the practice of treating a disease with minute doses of drugs that produce effects similar to that of the disease in a healthy person

inhalant any substance that easily forms a vapor under normal conditions

kava a mildly intoxicating drink, originated in Polynesia and made from the roots of the *Piper methysticum*

khat the small, serrated, bitter leaf of the *Catha edulis* tree; contains cathinone, a substance chemically and pharmacologically related to amphetamine. The leaf is chewed by certain peoples in the Red Sea area to relieve fatigue and depression

kif the name given to marijuana grown along the Moroccan Rif

koknar a widely abused drug in the Soviet Union; made from the stems and seedpods of opium poppies and common household chemicals. The drug is injected directly into the veins of the user and has caused widespread addiction and needle-borne hepatitis in Poland and Hungary

kompot a drug abused in Eastern Bloc countries; similar to koknar and made from opium poppy stalks and household chemicals

la santa rosa "the sacred rose." Marijuana grown near the Gulf of Mexico and chewed by certain Indian tribal groups in the area during religious rituals

LSD (lysergic acid diethylamide) a hallucinogenic drug derived from a fungus that grows on rye or from morning glory seeds

marijuana a psychoactive substance with the active ingredient THC; found in the crushed leaves, flowers, and branches of the hemp plant

MDMA known as "Ecstasy," methylenedioxymethamphetamine is a designer hallucinogen, (or a synthetic drug slightly different in chemical structure from an illicit natural hallucinogen)

mescaline a psychedelic drug found in the peyote cactus

methadone a drug that has been legally administered to heroin addicts to help them break their addiction; it is addictive and available in most countries by prescription only

methaqualone a prescription drug with the trade name Quaalude; used as a sedative

narcotic originally a group of drugs producing effects similar to morphine; often used to refer to any substance that sedates, has a depressant effect, and/or causes dependence

NBA nonbeverage alcohol; alcohol contained in hair tonics, mouthwash, and cleaning products consumed when there is no other alcohol available

opiates compounds from the milky juice of the poppy plant *Papaver somniferum*, including opium, morphine, codeine, and their derivatives (such as heroin)

PCP also called phencyclidine; an illicit drug used for its stimulating, depressing, and/or hallucinogenic effects

physical dependence an adaptation of the body to the presence of a drug such that its absence produces withdrawal symptoms

pitillo Bolivian coca paste cigarettes

psychological dependence a condition in which the drug user craves a drug to maintain a sense of well-being and feels discomfort when deprived of it

psychosis a severe mental illness characterized by hallucinations, mood disturbances, and loss of contact with reality

pulque a native Mexican drink made from the fermented sap of the maguey

sake a sweet traditional Japanese drink made from fermented rice

sedative a drug that produces calmness, relaxation, and sleep; barbiturates are considered sedatives

stimulant a drug that increases brain activity and produces the sensation of greater energy, euphoria, and increased alertness

thandai a drink made from bhang (the dried leaves of the cannabis plant), sugar, milk, spices, and seeds, considered a dietary supplement among the lower class in India

tolerance a decreased susceptibility to the effects of a drug as a result of its continued administration, resulting in the user's need to increase the drug dosage to achieve the effects experienced previously

tranquilizer an antianxiety drug that has calming and relaxing effects; Librium and Valium are tranquilizers

withdrawal the physiological and psychological effects of discontinued use of a drug

Index

PICTURE CREDITS

American Museum of Natural History/G. Ekholm: p. 76; AP/Wide World Photos: pp. 74, 90, 93, 123; Art Resource: pp. 80, 110; The Bettmann Archive: pp. 20, 55, 88, 115, 116, 120; Drug Enforcement Agency: p. 47; Stephen L. Feldman/Photo Researchers, Inc.: p. 28; Globe Photos: pp. 62, 85, 104, 106; Grunwald Center for Graphic Arts: p. 119; Herbert T. Hoover Collection: p. 25; Imtek Imagineering/Masterfile: cover; Irish Tourist Board: p. 50; National Library of Medicine: pp. 12, 38; New York Public Library Picture Collection: p. 22; Doris Pinney, Photo Library, Inc./Globe Photos: p. 18; Roy Pinney, Photo Library, Inc./Globe Photos: p. 96; Reuters/Bettmann Newsphotos: p. 87; John Robaton/United Nations Photos: pp. 34, 127; Jane Schreibman/United Nations Photos: p. 41; Maps by Mark Stein Studios: pp. 37, 52–53, 79, 82–83, 100, 103, 112, 134–135; Sudhakaran/United Nations Photos: p. 150; United Nations Photos: pp. 10, 64, 72, 125; UPI/Bettmann Newsphotos: pp. 8, 30, 31, 32, 42, 45, 56, 59, 60, 67, 69, 71, 73, 84, 98, 108, 130, 132, 137, 138, 140, 141, 143, 146, 148; Original Illustrations by Gary Tong: p. 48

Marc Kusinitz is a science writer currently working free-lance for *Clinician*, an international medical publication distributed to physicians. He is the author of *Drugs & the Arts* and *Celebrity Drug Use* in the ENCYCLOPEDIA OF PSYCHOACTIVE DRUGS published by Chelsea House. Dr. Kusinitz holds a masters degree in environmental health science from the University of Rhode Island and a doctorate in biology from New York University. He has served as news editor of the *New York State Journal of Medicine* and associate editor of *Scholastic Science World* and has written for *Technology Review, Science Digest,* and the *New York Times*.

Solomon H. Snyder, M.D., is Distinguished Service Professor of Neuroscience, Pharmacology and Psychiatry at The Johns Hopkins University School of Medicine. He has served as president of the Society for Neuroscience and in 1978 received the Albert Lasker Award in Medical Research. He has authored *Uses of Marijuana, Madness and the Brain, The Troubled Mind, Biological Aspects of Mental Disorder,* and edited *Perspective in Neuropharmacology: A Tribute to Julius Axelrod.* Professor Snyder was a research associate with Dr. Axelrod at the National Institutes of Health.

Barry L. Jacobs, Ph.D., is currently a professor in the program of neuroscience at Princeton University. Professor Jacobs is author of *Serotonin Neurotransmission and Behavior* and *Hallucinogens: Neurochemical, Behavioral and Clinical Perspectives.* He has written many journal articles in the field of neuroscience and contributed numerous chapters to books on behavior and brain science. He has been a member of several panels of the National Institute of Mental Health.

Joann Ellison Rodgers, M.S. (Columbia), became the Deputy Director of Public Affairs and Director of Media Relations for the Johns Hopkins Medical Institutions in Baltimore, Maryland, in 1984 after 18 years as an award-winning science journalist and widely read columnist for the Hearst newspapers. She is the author of *Drugs and Pain* in the ENCYCLOPEDIA OF PSYCHOACTIVE DRUGS SERIES 2, published by Chelsea House.